STRETCHING AND FLEXIBILITY EXERCISES FOR MEN:

FROM BEGINNERS TO GYM RATS, THIS IS YOUR ALL-INCLUSIVE GUIDE TO STRETCHING AND FLEXIBILITY FOR JOINT PAIN, INTRODUCTION TO EXERCISE, AND OTHER BENEFITS.

BENJAMIN LUCAS

CONTENTS

JOIN OUR COMMUNITY!

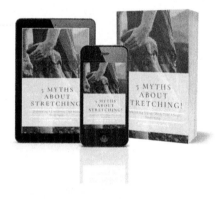

WOULD YOU LIKE A FREE GIFT?

Go to Benjaminlucasbooks.com and sign up. As a thank you we will give you "5 Myths About Stretching!".

This free gift will tell you 5 lies that are told in the stretching community and also will help you get on the right track on you stretching and flexibility journey.

INTRODUCTION

No matter where you are or what you're doing, you can always take a moment to stretch. You don't need to be a gymnast or a yogi either. For some reason, most people are afraid of stretching. It's nothing to be frightened of, as you'll soon discover. People think stretching is a painful ordeal, but that couldn't be further from the truth if you're doing it right.

Stretching does wonders for your posture. The more you stretch, the taller you stand, and the slimmer you look. With the right posture, your body will perform the way it's supposed to, and you'll find yourself breathing fully. If your posture isn't the best, chances are you've got some tight muscles that could use some loosening up. Now, it's easy to assume posture isn't a big deal. It's not like you're a royal, or you're having lunch with the Queen or something. However, bad posture goes beyond just not looking your best. It's caused by imbalances in your muscles that then lead to a misaligned skeleton.

Think of your skeleton as the frame on which the rest of you hangs. If that's out of alignment, you'll naturally look odd.

Again, it's more than just about looks. On the other side, one part of your body overcompensates for the shortcomings in muscular strength and flexibility. Pay attention to your body and how it feels the next time you carry your bag or briefcase in the same hand or on the same shoulder, or when you keep sleeping on the same side. It may seem like it's no big deal, but the imbalance you feel could be costing you energy, especially since you're not moving as efficiently as you could. Also, you can bet it's a contributing factor to your nagging back pain. This is where stretching could help you.

Stretching makes you nice and limber. Whether we like it or not, muscles tend to grow tighter and shorter with time. That's why the older you get, the less your range of motion becomes. If your muscle is always tight and short, then you don't expect it to perform as well as it should when contracted because it's been in a perpetually contracted state, leaving you open to injury. With stretching, you will improve your functional flexibility, which allows you to do your thing every day.

My name is Benjamin Lucas, I have been an amateur Muay Thai fighter for over 5 years. Beyond that, I have spent my entire life working out and in gyms. Anyone who works out in a gym can tell you that the most frustrating part of working out in a gym is the soreness that you feel from growing and training a specific muscle group. It becomes a pain to do regular day-to-day activities, you feel tired, fatigued, and miserable. It wasn't until I started stretching that I began to feel relief in my muscles from pain.

This wasn't what made me a full believer in stretching though. My true love for stretching came after an injury. I was at "Six Flags" with my brother and some friends. It was an amazing day, we got on all of the rides. When we were leaving my brother gave me a playful shrug. My brother is much bigger than me, so I jumped and threw my body into him. We were on the edge of the sidewalk and my right foot landed wrong. I tore a muscle behind the back of my knee.

For months there was this incessant pain that wouldn't stop. At first, I couldn't stand on it for more than a couple of hours without it hurting. I went to countless doctors, some refusing me an MRI due to cost, others recommending vitamins and supplements. I went to physical therapy for weeks and they would teach me stretches to help and this would work for a time, but after I stopped going to physical therapy the pain would slowly come back all over again. It wasn't until I started Muay Thai that I truly started to feel a change in my body.

Through my fight gym, we would have lots and lots of classes a week. When I first started Muay Thai it was the sorest that I had ever been. As a daily practice, in class, we always would stretch at the beginning and at the end of class. Not for too long but just enough to loosen the muscles a bit. I don't remember when, but one day my leg stopped hurting, and it hasn't hurt ever since. This is when I came to know that stretching is one of the most important things for athletes, but also it can be beneficial for everyone.

Stretching helps you when you need to bend, twist, turn, or do anything else, as your joints have a greater range of motion. This means you can engage in physical activities without being handicapped by an achy back, or tense muscles. When your functional flexibility isn't so great, even simple things like bending to pick up a pen cap can feel like moving mountains.

More stretching means fewer injuries. As you do your stretches, you'll find that you don't have as many injuries as you used to. If you do get injured, you'll notice that you recover faster, too. When you accidentally overstretch a muscle or strain your joints, stretching will help you immensely. Think of it as a very cheap and effective way to prevent bad stuff from happening to your body.

Stretching de-stresses, you. Stress happens. It's unavoidable, good in small doses, but absolutely terrible when that's your perpetual state of being. Being overly stressed will ruin your peace of mind and health. You know you're stressed when you find it hard to remember stuff, you're always on edge, and possibly even feeling depressed. When you get this way, stretching can help you find some relief by encouraging your muscles to relax. Add in some deep, conscious breathing, and you'll find your anxiety levels dropping like dead weight. Moving your body as slowly and deliberately as possible can cause your mind to enter a state of meditation, as you're focused less on your troubles and more on the feeling in each muscle. When you're meditating, you take a break from the stressors in your life, and that allows you to have a fresh perspective. That's how powerful stretching can be.

My goal with this book is to provide you with a platform to improve your quality of life and physical health through effective stretching. You'll learn about the benefits of stretching, the science behind it, and how to perform stretches safely. Discover proper breathing techniques and how to incorporate stretching into your daily routines.

Are you always on the move? Are you young and spry, or old and stiff? It doesn't matter anyway. You'll find different exercises that work for you no matter how old or young you are. You can do these stretches, and you'll thank yourself for picking this book up and putting in the time to make yourself feel better, younger, and more flexible.

You'll find this book is easy to grasp. The exercises are easy to follow, written in simple English, with hands-on instructions, so you don't feel lost at any point. Do you feel like you need to be a marathon runner or a fitness buff of some sort to gain benefits from stretching? That's not the case. You can begin as you are, and right away, you'll notice the benefits of giving your muscles a nice, luxurious stretch. If you don't have much experience with stretching, this book will walk you through it, so it feels as easy as pie.

The wonderful thing about stretching is that you really can perform it almost anytime and anywhere. Sitting at your desk too long? Get up and stretch. Feeling sluggish and stiff? Get up and stretch.

Stretching is one of the simplest and most rewarding exercises you can perform. A regular stretching routine can enhance your flexibility, muscle function, and circulation—all while calming your mind and improving your overall quality of life. Whether you're a couch potato, a fitness fanatic, or somewhere in between, you'll find that as you begin stretching regularly, you will move more fluidly and effortlessly.

We're going to address every body part that needs to get nice and limber so that you can reclaim your feeling of strength and youth once more and start to move in a more natural and freeing way. All you have to do is ensure you follow everything written here to the letter, don't overwork yourself, and most importantly, have fun.

ONE
SHOULD MEN STRETCH?

Stretching is a great tool for everyone, no matter your age or sex. Men, however, may not be so inclined to perform stretching exercises because of the following reasons:

Men are accustomed to being more active and are more in tune with their bodies than women. When they become inactive over time, they may not feel the need to exercise.

Men tend to exhibit less range of motion than women due to certain issues like weight training and competitive sports.

They are more likely to push through muscle pain and tightness when they exercise because of their competitive nature.

Men may not realize the importance of stretching because they spend less time sitting than women do.

WHY EVERY MAN SHOULD STRETCH FOR A BETTER WORKOUT

Even though male athletes may not be as prone to tightness as females, everyone can benefit from a good stretching routine. You don't have to be a fitness buff or even active in sports to see results from incorporating regular stretching into your lifestyle.

Stretching is especially important for men who work out or tend towards being more sedentary because it will improve their workout efficiency and reduce the chances of injuries. As men get older, they can experience issues like arthritis and joint pain due to a decrease in flexibility. Stretching allows them to bend easier and lift more comfortably.

Men who are over the age of 35 should really consider stretching as a good addition to their fitness routine because it helps keep their muscles functioning well. Not only is it a great muscle toner, but it builds strong, lean muscles.

Stretching is equally important for active people who want to take care of their bodies to continue doing sports without injury. When you stretch, you improve your agility and reduce the risk of getting injured during a workout.

Men tend to neglect their flexibility, which can develop over time as they get older. This issue can cause muscle tightness or stiffness that is extremely painful and can stop them from doing even simple activities like bending down to tie their shoes.

As men get older, they tend to put on a lot of weight, which puts more stress on the joints and muscles. Stretching can aid in weight loss and reduce stress when done in conjunction with other workouts.

A good stretch routine provides multiple benefits. From increased blood flow to increased flexibility, stretching provides a full-body workout that will improve your overall health and quality of life.

WHAT HAPPENS IF YOU STRETCH EVERYDAY

Stretching has many different benefits, from improved flexibility to reduced stress and injury risk. Even if you are currently active, you can still benefit from stretching even more by including it in your everyday routines, whether morning or evening. The more you stretch, the more benefits you will receive.

If you stretch every day, your flexibility will improve, your muscles will stay healthy and strong, and your body will be in a better position for any other type of exercise or athletic activity. If you are currently active and do not want to get less flexible as you age, holding stretches for five to ten seconds is recommended as it allows for maximum relaxation.

But, if you are an active individual and would like to see even more results, full stretches should be performed at least twice a day.

The goal of stretching is to achieve maximum flexibility. When held for a certain amount of time, the loosening of muscles during full stretches will allow muscles to relax fully in between exercises and activities without the wearer feeling overly stretched or uncomfortable.

Regular stretching helps increase your range of motion, which will help you avoid injuries. If you are on your feet all day, such as in a desk job or in the military, stretching before you come back to work will help prevent stiffness and muscle soreness.

Stretching helps people maintain flexibility throughout the day because it allows muscles to recuperate slowly. Even if you only stretch at the beginning of your day, even if it is only a few minutes, holding stretches longer than five seconds will allow your muscles to recuperate and prepare for another stretch.

TYPES OF RUNNING STRETCHES

Well, that is static stretching. Not all stretches are static stretches – there are dynamic stretches too. So, what's the difference? Dynamic stretches require motion, while static stretches are the ones where you just stand up, sit down, or stay in place and then stretch.

So does that mean we don't do static stretches at all?

Of course not; in fact, you need to do both types of stretches. Well, here's what you should do. After you have done your initial walk or trot to warm up your muscles, the next step is to do some dynamic stretches. After doing dynamic stretches, you can go on running.

Note that running, just like any kind of workout, will make your muscles really tight. Yes, they will be toned and primed, but they will feel tight – sometimes too tight. You will feel the tension in your legs; you may even get some imbalances after running a mile or so. Eventually, if you're not careful, you may develop unwanted injuries.

To prevent that from happening, you should give your legs, i.e., hip muscles, calves, hamstrings, quads, etc., some good stretching. The type of stretches you need to do post-run are static stretches.

Static stretches and dynamic stretches are important phases of anyone's running routine. You just can't do without them, and they are a big help to prevent different types of injuries.

BENEFITS OF DYNAMIC AND STATIC STRETCHING

Note that dynamic stretches help to loosen up your leg muscles, and they should be done before an actual run. These stretches get them prepped for the arduous task of flexing and extending over and over again just to propel your body forward.

It's a tough task, and dynamic stretches help to activate them – remember, they were in a slightly relaxed state before you warmed up with a little walking and trotting.

Static stretches should be done after your run. Tight

muscles should be stretched to help them relax. These stretches can also reduce muscle soreness and prevent injury. They also help lower your heart rate.

STRETCH OR DIE

Why Every Guy Should Be Stretching Post-Workout

Stretching can be performed to increase flexibility and range of motion, reduce fatigue and increase endurance, improve performance, prevent injury, and other benefits. Many different types of stretching are used.

There are numerous benefits of stretching; however, the following are a few examples:

Increase in flexibility: Stretching helps increase flexibility. A person must have enough flexibility in the tissues of their muscles to perform activities efficiently. Increased range of motion: Stretching helps increase the range of motion in joints.

Preventing injury: Stretching is useful since it lengthens the ligaments, tendons, and muscles. This helps them withstand a sudden force that may lead to an injury. It is believed that stretching can help prevent injuries to tendons as well as muscles that are caused due to repetitive movements.

Flexibility: Stretching helps increase a muscle or joint range of motion. This will enable the muscles to perform exercises with greater ease and speed, which in turn will improve performance.

Preventing muscle fatigue: Stretching can reduce the formation of adhesions between fibers, leading to decreased muscular capacity and increased fatigue. Adhesions are also commonly associated with injury. A person performing dynamic stretching post-training can help reduce this aspect of muscle fatigue and thus help prevent injuries caused by a lack of physical recovery.

The person should ensure that the stretches are done gradually. The right amount of time should be placed between each position to prevent injuries.

There are numerous benefits of stretching; however, the following are a few examples:

Reduces soreness: Stretching reduces muscle soreness when used after exercise or other physically taxing activities. Increases flexibility: Stretching increases flexibility and range of motion in muscles and joints, which helps prevent injuries when used prior to exercise.

THE IMPORTANCE OF STRETCHING

Stretching keeps the muscles flexible, strong, and healthy, and we need that flexibility to maintain a range of motion in the joints. Without it, the muscles shorten and become tight. Then, when you call on the muscles for activity, they are weak and unable to extend all the way. That puts you at risk for joint pain, strains, and muscle damage. Before a workout, do some dynamic stretching. This will help you warm up the muscle groups and improve your range of motion before you begin your workout.

Find time every day to stretch after a run or workout. Try static stretches, which are just as important as dynamic stretches. These static stretches should be performed with the muscles being held at the end of a range of motion until they become fully relaxed, and then you can gently massage and stretch the muscle again.

As with every subject you are new to, it's always recommended to understand the benefits and get yourself a bit more familiar with the subject. Don't worry; we'll get to the exercises when we've examined the importance of stretching. It's something we often neglect during our daily busy life, and therefore I'd like to create more awareness of this subject by handing out this book to the world. Every single movement you make, whether a significant or a tiny one, will require moving a part of your body towards a point where your joint has to be slightly increased. It will be called a stretching exercise.

I have listed down below some of the benefits of stretching for you.

- Great muscular flexibility.
- Reduced injuries and pains – Use light stretches if the pain prevails.
- Improved muscular strength, flexibility, and stamina – The benefit depends on the degree of how much stress you put on your muscle. For gaining more strength, medium or heavy stretches are recommended.
- Improved body posture and self-image.
- Prevention of back problems.

Having improved flexibility will bring great benefits, as you've noticed in the list above. It's a very common practice, especially in the Mediterranean region and parts of Asia. By practicing various stretching exercises regularly, you will help reduce the risk of getting injuries and muscle pains. As you become more experienced and your body becomes familiar with the exercises, you'll become a lot more efficient when performing physical activities. Should I have to explain all the great benefits and positive reactions to your body in just 4 words, I'd describe it as "improve quality of life." Ease in body movements will be provided for your everyday activities. Even the simplest tasks, such as bending over to pick up something off the floor, will be accomplished far more accessible, faster, better, and healthier when your body has improved flexibility.

I'd recommend for any person out there, whether you're an athlete or a beginner, to follow a stretching program. The great benefits you'll gain from it are worth the slight effort and time you've put into it. Recent research studies on various injuries have shown that people with low flexibility have a highly increased chance of muscle injuries. However, don't confuse this with performing stretching exercises before your physical activity. The flexibility required for a lower chance of getting injuries came from following a stretch training for a certain amount of weeks. By following stretch training, you will increase your body endurance and strength, and it has been reported that you'll increase your flexibility.

Before we get started, I'd like to hand out a couple of tips to you. The most important one is including the major muscle groups in your workout schedule. Personally, I've created a rule of thumb to perform at least two exercises per muscle group. It's always recommended to start light as part of your warm-up and slowly progress towards heavier exercises to avoid injuries.

After you've finished your workout routine, don't run towards the showers just yet. It is suggested to do a proper warm-up but also a cool-down once you've completed your routine. This can be done the same way as the warm-up. Should your muscles be sore after your exercises, try to use only light stretches ranging from two to three times. Should your muscle soreness or injury persist for several days, I recommend using light stretches only. It is very important to give your muscles enough rest to recover, instead of forcing them.

KNOW YOUR LIMITS

Now that we know the many great benefits that stretching has to offer, it is also important to know your limits and what to avoid. We'll start focusing on the primary part of any workout program, knowing your limits. Working out has to be something that you should enjoy and look forward to. If you don't find any pleasure in implementing it into your daily life, how are you supposed to stick to a habit you dislike?

It can be the first thing you do in the morning when you

wake up or in the evening when you finish your working shift. Times may come when you'll be experiencing slight muscle soreness while you're performing an exercise or the next day. This is all fine, but keep in mind that the pain shouldn't be a type of pain that prevents you from doing your normal physical activities.

The same theory goes for stretching. Stretching properly before, during, and after a workout session will definitely decrease the chances of obtaining some serious injuries and avoid muscle soreness and pains.

It is therefore essential to know your body limits. Stretching is an activity that should improve your body stamina rather than cause you pain. Stretching was invented to avoid pain and become more flexible. You might feel a small mild tension when you stretch, do not worry as this is just a temporary feeling from your body stiffness. If you feel pain beyond this, then you've overdone it, and it's necessary to lower the tense level of your exercises.

Should you feel pain during stretching, this means that your body has employed its defense mechanism – the stretch reflex. How exactly do you trigger your defense mechanism? When you're performing stretching exercises, you stretch your muscles towards the level where you start feeling "pain." Our bodies have evolved over the years and created safety measures to reduce the risk of harming your muscles and tendons with possible damage. The defense mechanism that we call the stretch reflex protects your muscles. There may come times when you are too excited to stretch your muscles and tendons beyond their limits. Luckily, our stretch reflex will try and prevent this from happening. Although we have a great mechanism, you should never try and force your body beyond the limits. You will risk causing serious damage to your muscle tissues, tendons, and ligaments.

WHY YOU SHOULD DO STRETCHES
EVERY DAY

1. Stress relief - Stretching is a great thing to do when you're feeling stressed out or having an anxiety attack. A great way to release your stress is to stretch your muscle tissues and hold them for a few seconds every time you feel stressed out. Try NOT to stretch your muscles excessively – this can cause unnecessary harm to your muscles and tendons.

2. Chronic pain relief - Should you experience pain for more than two weeks, it's suggested to start stretching daily. Stretching will increase your flexibility, thus increasing blood and oxygen flow to the muscle tissue and tendons. This sticks a little bit longer so that the stretch reflex can take effect, thus reducing possible damage to your muscles and tendons.

3. Improved blood circulation - The more flexible you are, the easier it is to move your body around. A great way to increase your flexibility level is by exercising regularly (minimum once a week). When you exercise your muscles, they will get warm and more flexible.

4. Injury prevention - Stretching is a must before exercising. You want your muscles and tendons to be warmed up before exercising. This way, they won't get damaged when you're exercising with high pressure.

5. Increased flexibility - Not only will you increase your flexibility level, but you will also prevent injuries. When you stretch your muscles and tendons after exercising, they'll be slightly stiff. You should try to gently stretch them as a way of loosening up the stiff muscles.

6. Weight loss - A great way to lose weight is by stretching daily. It increases the elasticity of your muscle tissues, which in turn allows them to lose weight without feeling extra fatigue (this is because the elasticity of your muscle tissues helps to store more usable energy).

TWO

BENEFITS OF STRETCHING

S tretching is a great way to increase your flexibility. A stretch is a technique in which you use your muscles and tendons to contract and lengthen muscles, releasing tension voluntarily. The purpose of stretching is to make it easier for the body's muscles to fight against gravity as they flex, bend, extend and twist. Stretching has been proven to be beneficial for our muscles and those who have been injured or suffered an injury (such as tendons). Stretching helps improve blood flow, circulation, and endurance throughout our bodies.

STRESS

Stretching will help us to relieve muscle stress. When stressed out, it is common to experience tension in our muscles. It is a normal stress response that allows us to perform at our best when we need to. Stretching will help us release the tension and make us calmer.

STRESS EFFECTS ON THE BODY

Stress is a physical and mental state that can be triggered by many things, most notably any stressful life event. When we are stressed out, our muscles are constricted, which inhibits blood flow. This can lead to a decrease in performance. The human body usually responds to stress by triggering the response of the "fight or flight" mechanism, which describes involuntary autonomic nervous system responses intended to protect us in situations where there is an immediate threat to our survival. Stress is often viewed as negative, but it can be positive, such as the excitement of a game or competition. When we feel stress during a game or competition, it is common for us to tense up and have knots in our muscles. However, if we can stretch the knots out during and after the game/competition, this will help us prevent injuries and improve our performance in the next game or competition.

LONG TERM EFFECTS OF STRESS ON THE BODY

The long-term effects of stress can cause many illnesses and disorders. Stress can lead to muscle tension, and it can even lead to fibromyalgia, a condition where the muscles are constantly tense and painful. When we are stressed out, our bodies stop producing enough serotonin and dopamine, which are hormones that affect mood. This leads to increased anxiety and depression, which is known as "stress" or "neuroticism." These are also known as "fight or flight" hormones. Stretching will help us release the tension in our muscles so that we can perform at our best during stressful situations. When we stretch our muscles, it will allow us to feel more relaxed and stress-free. This will allow us to perform even better when needed because of the improved blood flow, circulation, and endurance throughout the body.

Stress affects the entire body, including the Musculoskeletal system. When we are stressed out, our body will release stress hormones, and these hormones will cause the muscles to tense up and become stiffer. When this happens, our muscles aren't as flexible anymore, so we can feel stiffer when stressed out. This is also why it's really important to stretch our muscles before stress happens.

Stress also affects the Respiratory System and Cardiovascular systems. It is common for people to breathe more shallowly when stressed out. This makes the heart work harder to pump blood through the body, and as a result, the lungs have to work harder to supply oxygen to the blood being pumped through the body. This is why doctors suggest focusing on controlling our breathing when we are stressed out. Stretching our muscles can help us stretch out any tension we may have in our chest, and it can also help us take the deep breaths we need so that we don't feel as tense. Stretching will also help us better supply oxygen to our muscles and organs.

Stress can also affect the Digestive System. When we are stressed out, it is common for us to feel as though we are not able to digest food properly and that it comes out of our stomach in waves. There is usually more fluid in our bodies when we are stressed out, leading to indigestion. It is important to remember that stretching is an important tool to help navigate stress, and because of this, it can lead to overall positive effects on the body.

JOINT PAIN

When we are stressed out or have experienced an injury, our joints can take a lot of damage. The joints can become stiff, making it harder to bend and stretch them because there is more tension in our muscles.

CAN STRETCHING RELIEVE JOINT PAIN?

Stretching can significantly relieve joint pain if we stretch our joints in the same way it relieves pain in other areas of our body. For example, if we have a muscle pull or sprain, stretching our muscles will help them feel much more flexible. It will also relieve the stiffness that we feel and over time help the pain go away altogether. If we have chronic neck or back pain, then stretching out those muscles will hopefully strengthen them allowing us to get rid of the stiffness and the pain.

As far as men are concerned. We experience pain in all forms. A lot of us experience pain at work. We sit in chairs for hours from 9-5, have to lift things at home, and have to fix and carry things around our houses. All of these things can lead to immense amounts of pain. This is where I want to emphasize the importance of stretching. Stretching is a vital part of relieving the pain men experience from the workplace, home, and errands. Relieving those muscles and protecting your body is important in a long healthy life, regardless of whether you want to exercise often, or just want a long and successful career.

HOW DOES STRETCHING HELP JOINTS?

Stretching is a great way to strengthen and balance muscles and help us recover from injuries faster. Our joints don't work very hard, and we need to give our muscles time to get used to being stretched out. Give your body some time to heal before you start stretching again. If you are going to stretch out your joint pain, then it is recommended that you stretch a little bit right after or at the same time that you start taking pain relievers or pain killers.

DOES STRETCHING MAKE ARTHRITIS WORSE?

No, but it's not going to cure your arthritis. If you have arthritis, it's best to check with a doctor before doing any activity to see if you are at risk of making your arthritis worse. If you have Rheumatoid Arthritis, then stretching can make your condition much worse and even cause death in some cases.

HOW TO STRETCH YOUR JOINTS CORRECTLY

When we stretch our joints, it makes them stronger and more flexible, but stretching can sometimes hurt our joints or cause pain. If we do not warm up before stretching out our muscles, we will pull ourselves. So, we must stretch only after warming up by doing other activities that increase the blood flow to our muscles like walking or bicycling.

DOES ACTIVE STRETCHING HELP JOINT PAIN?

Yes and no, active stretching can help relieve joint pain if we do it right. Active stretching can be a great way to get more flexibility into our joints, but it can also harm us. If you have arthritis, you should ask your doctor if it is safe for you to do any stretching before you try it out. Many people are getting injuries doing active stretches because they are not following the correct procedures for warming up or cooling down.

One of the important things to remember with stretching is that the body works in tandem with each part of it. What I mean by that is, let's say you have been experiencing long-term pain in your leg. You would think that you just should stretch out just that leg, spending more time on the part that is hurting. This is false however, you should stretch out both legs, and even your lower back. The body is so amazing that strengthening some parts of your body can help you to relieve pain in other parts.

SEX LIFE

As if stretching didn't have enough benefits for men, it also helps in the bedroom. Yes, stretching also can help improve your sex life. Because stretching can help to increase blood flow and circulation, it can help increase energy levels and stamina. This is a direct correlation to lasting longer in the bedroom.

What people tend not to realize, is the effect that stress, tension, or anxiety can have on our libido. It directly and dramatically affects it. When we stretch, we can unwind and start to put some of those stressors away. This helps us to be the best partners that we can be inside of the bedroom.

This can also help to make sex a lot more exciting for you and your partner. It is a saying said time and time again, but the saying is that we are at the mercy of our bodies. Simply means that we can only do what our body allows us to do. Stretching makes you more flexible and limber, and this new flexibility can reignite your sex life with your partner. Have you seen a position that you are interested in trying but couldn't try before? Now your body can try it. Does it hurt to hold a specific position for more than a short amount of time? Your body has become more durable and your muscles have started to develop strength. This completely revitalizes sex with your partner and can turn it into a place of fun and experimentation.

Finally, and this is the big one. You know, the one that we don't like to talk about as men, Erectile Dysfunction. Erectile Dysfunction is something that happens in a lot of men. There are thousands of men who cannot get erections or cannot sustain them. An erection happens because of blood flow, therefore poor blood flow can be a big cause of why a man isn't getting the desired erection to perform at their desired level. Stretching can help to keep the blood flowing and as a result, help you with your arousal and erections. Take care of your body and it will take care of you. Or in this case, help you take care of someone else's.

BUILDING CONFIDENCE IN YOUR BODY/ A GOOD START TO GETTING ACTIVE

Stretching can be a great way to build confidence in your body. When we stretch our bodies, it makes us feel more powerful and confident because we use our bodies to their full potential. This will allow us to be more active and not get as tired or hurt as easily when we do physically demanding activities.

We can also gain confidence in our bodies by doing regular workouts or, better yet, yoga classes. Yoga is a great way to gain more power and confidence in your body because it allows us to get our bodies in shape while learning inner peace and balance.

When we have more confidence in ourselves, it will make us much more active because we will be more comfortable with using our bodies. This allows us to be more physically active without worrying about getting tired or hurting ourselves.

In addition, it is an amazing way to start getting active. I can imagine it for you. A man who has decided to start working out. You want to be much more active this year. You tell yourself that you are going to go to the gym. You buy a membership, and you head to the gym. Immediately you are overwhelmed by all of the machines, weights, and contraptions that you know you have no idea how to use. Men and women who seem confident and comfortable in their bodies while you are just starting. Stretching is an amazing way to start getting active. Through utilizing a full stretch routine you are getting used to actively using your body, and after a certain amount of time, you will be able and confident enough to hit the weights and machines. Just as confidently as everyone else.

WHAT IS THE BEST WAY TO STRETCH?

There are a lot of different ways to stretch our muscles and joints. The best way to stretch is to do stretching exercises that work multiple parts of the body at one time. For example, if we wanted to stretch the hip flexors, we would start thereby:

bending and lifting one leg while encouraging the other leg to straighten up as well.

If you haven't ever moved your body and want to start, stretching is a great way to do it because it doesn't require a lot of activity. Stretch any time of the day, and by doing it, you are building confidence in your body. Knowing a few yoga poses can also give you a good way to stretch out your muscles and bend your joints

THREE
HOW TO START

The way to train is to make sure that you are using your muscles and joints in the right way. It is best to start by doing activities that don't require a lot of exertion, such as walking or light hiking. This will help your body get used to moving with ease. It is also a good idea to start with some stretching techniques as well because it also builds confidence in your body.

WHERE TO START

Being aware of the best stretching method for your body is a great asset to have. This allows you to maintain great flexibility without even having to warm up. Athletes especially need to have such flexibility to demonstrate a technique immediately when it is required. Lacking this ability will indicate that your stretching method's use is incorrect, or you are chronically fatigued. In some cases, in a worst-case scenario, you could be dealing with both.

Should you be one of the persons who have this flexibility, bear in mind not to get too confident. If you are familiar and experienced with sports, you will not necessarily always have to do a complete set of stretching before doing a few full ranges of motion moves without a warm-up; however, you should never overdo it. Many sports involve sudden twisting or bending of the trunk, such as football, rugby, basketball, and kickboxing. Without warming up your muscles, this will result in back pain. The back is wrapped in deep layers of muscles. The larger and deeper the mass of your muscles is, the longer it takes to warm them up. Warming them up before doing your workout will result in recovery afterward.

One of the most straightforward athletic training tasks is developing great flexibility. One can reach an exceptional level with very little time and effort. With rational training, your flexibility will improve from day to day. We have examined the most common mistakes which withhold most people who spend days and weeks in the gym without getting better results.

Applying the methodology, you will find in this book will improve your results and prevent you from making any of the previously discussed mistakes. If you follow the instructions in the letter, you will have a very small chance to obtain muscle injuries and pain.

You will find many methods for improving flexibility out there; I have tried to sum up the safest and most efficient ways for you. Everybody asks for a different kind of combination or method. This highly depends on the current shape you are in. I will try to guide you towards the best possible methods for you.

DYNAMIC STRETCHING

One of the very good ways of stretching is dynamic stretching. A quick way of explaining it would be; to increase the reach and speed of your movements. Always perform your exercises in sets of 8 to 10 repetitions. Should you feel tired after a few sets, stop immediately. Fatigue will cause a decrease in the amplitude of your movements. It is recommended to only exercise the number of repetitions that you can do without diminishing your range of motion. If you do more repetitions than your body allows, you will more than likely lose some of your flexibility. After you have reached the maximum range of motion in a joint, you should stop with this particular movement in a direction. Even if you can maintain your current maximum range of motion, it is not advised to force it.

Dynamic stretches are often confused with static stretches. Dynamic stretches do not involve stopping and holding your stretched position. Dynamic stretching is supposed to increase your dynamic flexibility. Once your body is in motion, the speed of your movements and range will increase. These results are obtained by practicing dynamic stretches.

Dynamic stretching is also confused with ballistic stretching. Ballistic stretches are all about using the momentum of a moving body part or limb to forcibly and abruptly increase the range or speed of the motion. Unlike dynamic and static movements, a ballistic movement cannot be corrected or adjusted once it's started. In many cases, ballistic or bounce stretches will result in immediate as well as residual pain.

Now that you have learned the differences, you will probably understand that dynamic stretching is very different from ballistic or static stretching. There are no bobbling, bouncing, or jerky movements with dynamic stretching. The movements are controlled thoroughly even though they can be quite fast. As opposed to ballistic stretching, the dynamic stretches are not sudden and abrupt.

The arm swings, which we have used previously as an example, can practically be performed with control through the whole range of movement or with no control over a substantial part of the movement as soon as the stretch takes place.

STATIC STRETCHING

Most people who read this are most likely aware of what static stretching is. It involves moving your body into a stretch and then holding it there through the tension of your muscles. This is the stretch you will see people doing most commonly. When you tense your muscles harder, you may notice that you will feel less resistance from your stretched muscles.

There is a difference between doing static active stretches and static passive stretches. Passive stretching involves relaxing your body into a stretch and holding it there by your body weight or by external weights. A very good way to use passive stretches is to relieve cramps in overstimulated muscles. If you have spasms occurring in your muscles that are recovering after an injury or soreness, then you should also be using mainly static stretches. However, should you have sore muscles at that particular time, you may further damage them. When your muscles feel sore, it is a sign to give them rest as you have most likely used them actively. It is very important to find the right balance to avoid any injury that could have been avoided by giving the muscles enough rest. Should you not be entirely sure whether your muscles are sore or not, a safe method is to stretch very lightly.

Always keep in mind that you should not be exercising or stretching after or while being injured. It is advised to wait until you have healed sufficiently, and in case you are dealing with a serious injury, you should ask for advice from your doctor.

I've found that stretching passively within 30 seconds is the most effective. There's no need to do this multiple times per day unless you have a muscle injury or muscle soreness – then I would advise you to take more rest as needed.

BALLISTIC STRETCHING

Last but not least, we will get more involved with Ballistic stretching. The reason why there are so many different types of stretching is simply that performing one of them alone isn't enough. Ideally, you'd want to perform all the different stretching exercises to get the best results for your flexibility. It is therefore important to also understand Ballistic stretching and use them whenever possible.

While your muscles are fatigued, it may happen that your static flexibility will increase. You should consider doing more static stretches whenever this happens instead of near the end of your routine. However, Ballistic stretching is undoubtedly the fastest way to develop passive flexibility. It will improve that, but it also improves active flexibility and strength in various places. If you are a young reader, it is not recommended to do Ballistic stretching. I'd highly recommend waiting until your body has fully grown and your muscles are at their maximum strength before performing Ballistic stretching exercises. Not only is this important for children or young adults, but it is also meant for the people out there who have neglected training for a while. Don't underestimate the harm that Ballistic exercises can do to your body if done improperly.

If you feel like that person could be you, then please start with the basic stretching exercises first. A very good and safe way to increase your flexibility and strength is to execute a high amount of light repetitions of a certain exercise. But remember to not rush through them; you should always gently perform them in full-body range motion.

I've always been aiming to work on a certain muscle group 2 to 3 times per week. Do take note that the amount of strength exercises also depends on your body and muscle's reaction to them. It could happen that you've intensively worked on your legs during the previous day, and now those muscles are slightly sore. This means you were a little bit too excited and you should give them rest for now. Vice versa, this also goes for not getting muscle soreness together with poor progress; this means that you should exercise a bit more often or increase the weights.

Do not be afraid to make mistakes, be self-observant. The only way to learn how much and often you can increase your resistance and the frequency of your workout without getting sore muscles is trial and error. Whenever you obtain a minor injury, that tells you that you've lost strength and the particular muscles are a bit tense and short. If you're on your first day after an intense workout with muscle soreness, be ready because it will be worse on the second day. As stated before, never try and force your body over an injury or muscle soreness, this will not improve your flexibility, but it will most likely only get worse.

It's a question that I get many times, and it's always hard to measure. The question "how long would I need to give my muscles rest?". Frankly, only you could know. It's something that you have to experience, and as time goes by, you will get more familiar with the limits that your body has. Whenever you've obtained a level of muscle soreness, simply "test" your body. Meaning, that you have to see and test for yourself what kind of reaction your body and muscles will give you once you start performing a particular stretch. Whenever you feel that your body is still too weak and not ready for them, just stop and try the next day again.

Next up, I will explain three different methods of doing Ballistic stretches.

FIRST METHOD

A method that I prefer is stretching your muscles and waiting for a couple of seconds. How long should you wait? Just a moment so that you give your body enough time to adjust the length of your muscles. You'll know when you've held the stretch long enough by doing the same stretch again. You should start noticing a slight increase in your range. This should be done over and over again until you simply cannot stretch further anymore. Now, once you've done the first part and you've reached your stretching limit, you should start with short, strong tensions, followed by a short but quick relaxation, and immediately stretch again. Try to hold the last tension for at least 30 seconds and preferably longer.

SECOND METHOD

The second method can be slightly difficult and will probably take some practice before you truly master it. You should aim for the maximum once you're in a stretching position. Now that you've maneuvered yourself in a somewhat uncomfortable position, you have to hold this uncomfortable position a little bit more until you reach muscle spasms.

When your muscle starts to spasm, decrease the stretch for a moment. Once the spasms stop, increase and tense your muscles again until you reach the spasms. What's important is to hold the last tension for at least 5 minutes.

THIRD METHOD

The third and last method is the one I have used the most to get the best results. Stretch the muscles and tense them immediately for 3 short seconds, followed by a short moment of relaxation. I recommend staying in the preferred period of 1 to 5 seconds and then stretching the muscle again. Before stretching, try to maximally tense the muscles about to be stretched for a couple of seconds, followed by a relaxation of 1 to 5 seconds, then stretch the muscles again when you hit the near-maximal stretch, tense for a couple of seconds to trigger the lower resistance to a stretch and the stretch reflex.

Now try to increase the stretch until your limit. Be cautious when doing this.

It is a non-stop experiment to determine the tension's duration and strength, which gives you the best and most stretch upon relaxation. Suggested for the best effects during a stretch is to tense the muscles opposing the stretched ones. Bear in mind that this suggestion cannot be made for every stretch, such as standing stretches for the legs.

Gently increase the period while holding the tension to 30 seconds after several weeks of working out. Recommended is to take a minute of rest when you have reached the 30 seconds goal and repeat the same stretch. Try aiming for 3 times when doing this per workout.

When performing the previously described method, try to focus on strength gains when you find yourself in a certain stretched position. Whenever you feel that you're not able to increase the stretch anymore, continue by tensing your muscles. This will result in a greater stretch over time. A simple way to increase the tension of a muscle at any given length is to put extra weight on it. If you are doing leg splits, try not to support yourself with the help of your arms.

Whichever method you choose for Ballistic stretching, try to breathe naturally with deep and calm abdominal breaths when doing the stretches. Inhale before tensing and exhale or hold your breath during the maximal tension. Make sure to inhale at the beginning of relaxation and, if possible, exhale with further relaxation and stretch. Should you tense much longer than your normal exhalation, it is perfectly fine to inhale and exhale several times during the tension. There are positions where it may not be possible or convenient to exhale while relaxing and increase the tension's stretch. If you find yourself in this position, try to inhale during relaxation and stretching.

Choosing the preferred and best Ballistic stretches for your body will highly depend on the form of the movements in which you need a greater range of motion. Which one you should start with will depend on the muscle group you feel is the first obstacle. Which one feels the stiffest or the tightest? Is there pain anywhere? Do you want specific flexibility in a part of your body? There is no right or wrong way to start with your individual Ballistic stretches program. For example, if you would like to bring your outstretched arms behind your back while holding a stick in a narrow grip, the first resistance may come from your elbow flexors. This will tell you that you should stretch your elbow flexors first.

BUILDING A ROUTINE

When it comes to our bodies, any type of movement is good. It helps our overall bodily functions and promotes stronger and more durable muscles. It is quite easy to conclude that one doesn't need to make time for exercise in our daily lives explicitly, and once reaching a certain age in life, this is the number one thing to avoid. Our bodies decay if not in motion, and even if we are in motion, that might not always mean that the decay halts. But, with the help of a daily stretching routine, be it 10 minutes or 30 minutes a day, it all adds up over time.

If we assume that it takes roughly 21 days to break a habit, then the alternative must also be true: It only takes 21 days to create a habit. Whether you are 18, 55, or older, stretching and the improvement of your body is a great habit to pick up. Although the results might not be what we expect them to be, it is important to remember that the consistent repetition of a habit is what delivers long-term results.

THE BENEFITS OF REGULAR STRETCHING

Regular stretching helps us build up muscle strength, flexibility, and endurance. It helps our muscles contract and lengthens in a controlled way. It also helps us develop our core muscles which are vital to most of our movements.

1. Stress relief - Stretching helps us reduce stress by moving our muscles and joints through their full range of motion. This is because stretching contracts our muscles and causes them to relax. We can use this to help relieve pain, muscle tension, soreness, and stiffness in our bodies.

2. Increased flexibility - Stretching helps us increase our flexibility because our joints can expand and contract. Stretching is also safe for your joints because it increases blood flow to them. This is vital for the health of our joints because it provides nutrition that keeps them healthy and strong.

3. Better posture - Stretching can help us maintain good posture because it keeps our bodies straight. This is especially important if you are sitting a lot throughout your day. While sitting, our muscles and joints become stiff, causing our posture to become poor and causing pain in our lower back, neck, and shoulders.

4. Balance - When we stretch our body parts correctly, it will also help us develop balance because we can keep all parts of the body in balance as we stretch out each one. The correct way to stretch is to allow our muscles and joints to stretch out fully before we finally end the stretching.

5. Increased rebound - Stretching can also help us develop greater flexibility and better rebound because we can maintain good form by stretching our muscles and joints. Also, when we do a good job of stretching, it will help increase the amount of force that we can apply when performing an activity.

BEST PRACTICES

If you are one of the many people out there who are not getting the results you want from your exercise routine, this is most likely to do with your muscle groups being too stiff. When one muscle group is stiff, it will prevent others from improving and progressing. As stated previously, doing just static stretches where you hold your position is not necessarily the most effective approach to increase your flexibility. It involves contracting one muscle group while stretching the other. This triggers a muscular reflex that will increase your range of motion and deepen the stretch. As with all the other stretches, it does not have to take an hour per day of your time.

After your regular workout program, I have listed 6 stretches; try to do them slowly after every workout session. You will see improvement in your flexibility in just weeks; it will also improve both your strength and endurance in the same amount of time.

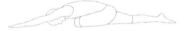

ACTIVE PIGEON STRETCH

Muscles: The Piriformis

GOOD FOR: Hip flexors, opening the hips, while working the lower back.

INSTRUCTIONS

1. Begin in a full push-up position, palms aligned under shoulders.
2. Place the left knee on the floor near the shoulder with the left heel by the right hip.
3. Lower down to the forearms and bring the right leg down with the top of the foot on the floor (not shown).
4. Keep your chest lifted to the wall in front of you, gazing down.
5. If you're more flexible, bring your chest down to the floor and extend your arms in front of you.
6. Pull the navel in toward the spine and tighten your pelvic-floor muscles; contract the right side of your glutes.
7. Curl right toes under while pressing the ball of your foot into the floor, pushing through your heel.
8. Bend knee to floor and release; do 5 reps total, then switch sides and repeat.

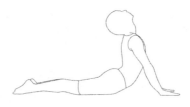

MODIFIED COBRA

Muscles: Abdominals

GOOD FOR: Stretching out the lower back, as well as chest, arms and abs.

· · ·

INSTRUCTIONS

1. Lie face down on the floor with your thumbs directly under the shoulders, legs extended with the tops of your feet on the floor.
2. Tighten your pelvic floor, and tuck your hips downward as you squeeze your glutes.
3. Press the shoulders down and away from your ears.
4. Push through your thumbs and index your fingers as you raise your chest towards the wall in front of you.
5. Relax and repeat.
6. Do 5 repetitions total.

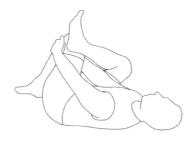

HAMSTRING STRETCH

Muscles: Hamstrings

GOOD FOR: Improve posture, increase flexibility, and loosening hip.

INSTRUCTIONS

1. Lie down face-up on the floor with your legs extended and feet flexed.
2. Bend your right knee to the chest and interlace your fingers behind the hamstrings as close to your groin as possible; gaze at your chest and keep your chin down and neck long.
3. Tighten your pelvic floor muscles and extend your leg, pushing through the heel and contracting quads.
4. Return to start and repeat; do 5 repetitions.
5. Repeat, turning the thigh outward for 5 repetitions.
6. Rest and repeat, turning the thigh inward for 5 repetitions.
7. Switch legs; repeat the series for a total of 15 repetitions on each leg.

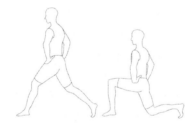

SPLIT SQUAT

Muscles: Quads, Calves

GOOD FOR: Strength development of the lower legs.

INSTRUCTIONS

1. Stand with your feet hip-width apart.
2. Step your right foot about 12 inches in front.
3. Curl the toes of your left leg; keep your weight equally between both feet. Interlace your fingers, placing your hands under the ribs; press the shoulders down away from your ears.
4. Tighten your pelvic floor muscles; tuck your pelvis under and squeeze your glutes.
5. Slowly bend both knees, coming down in 3 counts; feel the stretch along with the left quad.
6. Press into the floor to rise back to start in 3 counts.
7. Do 5 repetitions; switch legs and repeat.

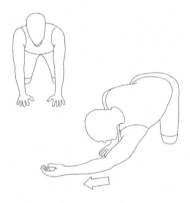

QUADRUPED STRETCH

Muscles: Shoulders

GOOD FOR: hip and shoulder loosening. This stretch will work everything from the shoulder to the oblique.

· · ·

INSTRUCTIONS

1. Kneel on all fours with your wrists aligned under the shoulders and knees under the hips.
2. Bring your forehead toward the floor and slide the pinkie edge of your left hand along the floor in front of you; keep your right palm flat on the floor.
3. Press the shoulders down away from your ears and squeeze your glutes.
4. Return to the starting position by pushing down on your right palm and sliding your left hand back toward your shoulders.
5. Do 5 repetitions; switch sides and repeat.

WHEN FINDING YOUR ROUTINE

Here are some tips to make your program last:

Your exercise routine is only as effective as your consistency. This means that no matter how great of a routine you follow, it fails if you do not stick to it.

There is a time and place for intensity, but in the beginning, you have to be able to stick with a program, and that means not skipping workouts or getting frustrated because your body is not already where you want it to be.

There will be times when you are not familiar with a certain exercise, and you have to be willing to ask someone for help.

- You might have to come up with excuses to get your workout in early in the morning, late at night, or during your lunch break. If you can't find the time, then change what you are doing so that it creates a time open for your exercise plan.

- You will find it easier if you work out with someone else.

Beginning a daily stretch routine is always a good idea. We have our bodies for only one life, and it's about time we gave them the attention they deserve. Make your exercise routine and stick to it if you want to get the body you desire.

- If you change your routine, which happens from time to time, just remember that the whole point is consistency in your exercise program. Be consistent in your lifelong commitment to fitness, and you will see results.

Stretching exercises:

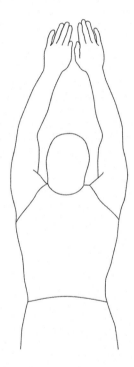

OVERHEAD STRETCH

Muscles: Chest, Shoulders, Triceps, Lats, Front Of Neck.

GOOD FOR: Working shoulders and the whole of your back.

. . .

INSTRUCTIONS

1. Standing with feet about hip-width apart, raise both arms above your head.
2. Reach your fingers, hands, and arms up as if you are trying to touch the ceiling. Take a deep breath in and then exhale.
3. If comfortable, look up and point your chin straight in front of you. Deep breath and exhale. If you have any neck pain or neck issues, skip this step.
4. With hands still raised, slightly bend the upper body backward and hold for 2 or 3 seconds, then return to standing straight.
5. Lower arms back down to sides.
6. Repeat the stretch two or three times.

Take Note:

• This can be done seated if you are unsteady on your feet or if you have any vertigo or balance issues.

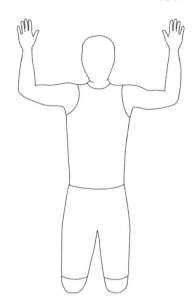

CACTUS ARMS

Muscles: Front of The Shoulder, Chest.

GOOD FOR: Building strength in the arms and chest.

INSTRUCTIONS

1. From a standing or seated position, raise arms overhead and then lower to bend at the elbow to form 90-degree angles, palms facing forward. Your arms should form a cactus or football goal post shape.
2. With your arms still raised and bent, push your chest forward as you push your arms slightly backward. Take a deep breath, then exhale and bring your chest and arms back to normal.
3. Repeat two or three times.

Take Note:

• Protect your lower back if you are standing or sitting by not arching your lower back while doing this stretch. If you find you are arching, you can do this stretch lying on your back and taking care to keep your lower back pressed to the floor.

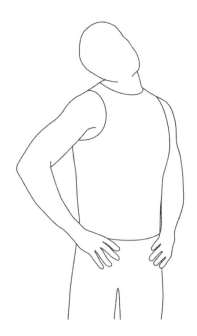

NECK ROLL STRETCH

Areas Stretched: Back And Sides Of Neck, Trapezius.

GOOD FOR: Loosening the Levator Scapulae.

INSTRUCTIONS

1. From a standing or seated position, look straight ahead. Slowly tilt your head to the left as if your left ear was trying to touch the top of your left shoulder. Be sure your shoulders do not hunch up! Keep them relaxed and down. Take a deep breath in and then exhale.
2. Slowly roll your head down to point your chin towards your chest. Remember to keep the shoulders relaxed. Deep breath in and then exhale.
3. Roll your head to the right. Your right ear should be facing down as if to touch the top of your right shoulder. Deep breath in and then exhale. Slowly bring the head back to a neutral, upright position. You can use your hands to help your head come back upright gently.
4. Repeat two or three times. You can alternate sides by starting with the right side first.

Take Note:

•Never tilt your head back while doing neck rolls. This puts a lot of unnecessary compression on your neck and spine.

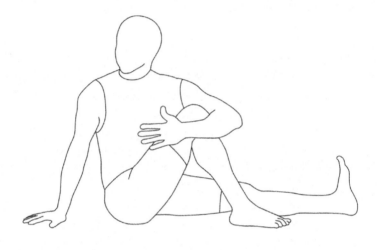

SEATED SPINAL TWIST

Areas Stretched: Entire Back, Upper Glutes.

GOOD FOR: Loosening tension in spine and chest.

INSTRUCTIONS

1. Sitting on the floor cross-legged, sit up tall and gently twist your upper body to the right. Place your left hand on your right knee and your right hand on the floor behind you.
2. If you can look to the back over your right shoulder. If not, keep your head relaxed and look ahead or down. Take a deep breath in, then exhale.
3. Return your upper body and head back to the front. Take a deep breath in, then exhale.
4. Change the cross of your legs, now putting the other leg in front.
5. Sit up tall and gently twist your upper body to the left. Place your right hand on your left knee and your left hand on the floor behind you.
6. Look to the back over your left shoulder, if possible. Otherwise, relax your neck and look ahead or down. Take a deep breath in, and then exhale.
7. Return your upper body and head back to the front. Repeat the stretch two or three more times.

Take Note:

•Keep both glutes firmly on the ground. If one side is lifting, you are twisting too far. Only twist as far as you are comfortable.

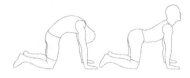

CAT COW POSE

Muscles: Upper Back, Mid Back, Back Of Neck, Shoulders.

GOOD FOR: Stretches and exercises like this are amazing for fixing and relegating posture by movement of the spine.

INSTRUCTIONS

1. Get on your hands and knees on the floor. Your hands should be directly under your shoulders and your knees directly under your hips. Your back should be neutral and roughly parallel to the floor.
2. Take a deep breath and inhale while gently lifting your head and your tailbone. Your back will arch slightly, and your belly will hang and be loose. This is called the cow stretch.
3. While exhaling, gently lower your chin towards your chest as you round your upper back towards the ceiling. Keep your tailbone, and your abdominals tucked in but don't clench them. This portion is called the cat stretch.
4. Repeat the cow and cat stretches slowly, flowing several times from one to the other.

Take Note:

•Keep your shoulders away from your ears and relaxed while doing this stretch. There should not be any tension in your neck or shoulders.

•If your wrists cannot support you, a variation of this stretch can be done seated. Sit cross-legged and place your hands on your knees while doing the cat and cow stretches.

FOUR
CHAPTER 4 ARMS

The arms, along with the wrists and hands, are the versatile workhorses of the body—performing feats of physical strength and detailed maneuvers. Our arms drive us, they hold groceries, they lift weights and hold babies. They are absolutely essential. Here are some stretches that you can use to keep your arms functioning at their best capabilities.

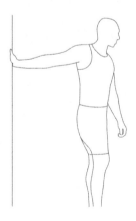

WALL-ASSISTED BICEP STRETCH

AFFECTED AREAS

Shoulders: deltoids

Chest: upper pectorals

Upper arms: biceps

Forearms

GOOD FOR:

This simple wall-assisted stretch lengthens the muscles along your chest, down your arms, and into your wrists. Find soothing relief from tight chest muscles and stiff shoulders and arms.

For a more intense opening along the back of your neck, slowly turn your head away from the wall to look toward the opposite shoulder.

Root down through your legs and engage your core muscles so that your weight is fully supported from your center. Try not to tense up your shoulders.

TYPE: STATIC, PASSIVE

INSTRUCTIONS

1. Stand with your right side about a foot away from a wall.
2. Step your left foot forward into an open stance.
3. Extend your right arm to shoulder height, and rest the palm of your hand on the wall above you.
4. Keeping contact with the wall, allow your right arm to slowly circle back and down behind you, bringing your hand to rest just below shoulder height.
5. Open your chest and slightly bend your left knee, shifting your weight several inches forward.
6. Inhale and exhale deeply as you hold here for 15 to 30 seconds.
7. Switch sides and repeat three times on each arm.

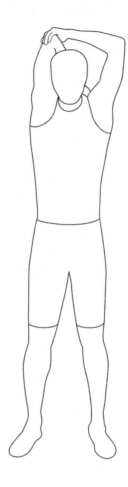

TRICEP STRETCH

AFFECTED AREAS

Upper arms: triceps, biceps

Shoulders: deltoids

GOOD FOR:

Counterbalance the downward pull of gravity on your arms by lifting your arms overhead and lengthening the sides of your body. You'll be able to loosen the area along the back of your arms as well as find some solace from tight shoulders.

Throw in a towel to ramp up this stretch. Grab one end of a rolled-up towel with your raised arm. Bring your opposite hand to your lower back and gently pull on the towel for 15 to 30 seconds.

Try to engage your core muscles and open your chest as you perform this exercise. Keep your back straight throughout.

TYPE: STATIC

INSTRUCTIONS

1. Find a comfortable stance or a supported seated position.
2. Raise your left arm straight up along your left ear.
3. Turn your arm inward so that your palm is facing behind you.
4. Bring your right hand up to support your left elbow as you slowly bend your left elbow, reaching your palm to the back of your left shoulder.
5. Use your right hand to gently press your left elbow up and back for a stretch. Hold for 20 seconds at the top of the move and breathe.
6. Repeat three to four times.

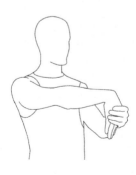

WRIST FLEXION

AFFECTED AREAS

Upper arms: biceps

Forearms: pronators, extensors, wrist flexors

GOOD FOR:

If your daily routine involves a lot of work with your hands or you have a hobby such as weight lifting, tennis, cooking, sewing, or gardening, this simple dynamic stretch will provide extensive relief through your wrists, forearms, and fingers.

Intensify the stretch by curling your extended fingers into a downward-facing fist. While keeping light pressure on the back of your wrist with your supporting hand, gently pull your fist down and away from your wrist.

The shoulder of the extended arm will naturally want to lift, but try to keep both shoulders square and relaxed. Imagine pulling your shoulder blades down your back.

TYPE: STATIC, PASSIVE

INSTRUCTIONS

1. Begin either standing or seated, and extend your left arm straight out in front of you.
2. Press your left fingers and thumb together, and flex your wrist downward, pointing your fingers toward the floor.
3. With your right hand, gently press your left fingers bringing them closer into your body.
4. Hold for 15 to 30 seconds, and repeat three to four times.

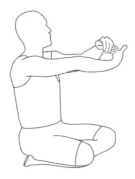

WRIST EXTENSION

AFFECTED AREAS

Forearms: pronators, extensors, wrist flexors

GOOD FOR:

Your wrists and hands control and facilitate multiple daily tasks. Additionally, with the onset of texting, your hands rarely get a break for very long. Ease away painful wrist tension and hand cramping with this stretch—a little extension goes a long way.

For an additional challenge, hold your arm in place, and slowly bend and straighten your extended elbow while keeping light pressure on your palm with the supporting hand.

It might surprise you how much of the stretch you feel with this simple move. You need only apply light pressure from your supporting hand to achieve a maximum stretch.

TYPE: STATIC, PASSIVE

INSTRUCTIONS

1. Begin seated or standing, and extend your right arm straight out in front of you, palm facing down.
2. Press your right fingers and thumb together, and pivot your wrist upward, pointing your fingers toward the ceiling.
3. Stretch from the base of your wrist as you bring your left hand to your right fingers.
4. With your left hand, gently press your right fingers back.
5. Hold for 15 to 30 seconds, and repeat three times on each wrist.

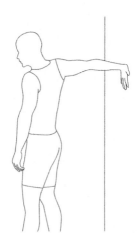

WALL-ASSISTED FOREARM STRETCH

AFFECTED AREAS

Upper arms: biceps

Forearms: pronators, extensors, wrist flexors

GOOD FOR:

This highly effective stretch calls for you to turn your arm outward, exposing your inner forearm up to the ceiling while bringing your wrist into full extension. With the support of the wall, this stretch is ideal for anyone who needs a little extra help with balance.

Tilt your head away from the wall to feel more lengthening through your upper arm, shoulder, and neck.

Try to open your fingers as wide as you can while your palm is in contact with the wall. This will assure an even stretch through your hand and fingers.

TYPE: STATIC, PASSIVE
INSTRUCTIONS

1. Stand with your right side positioned about arm's distance from a sturdy wall.
2. Bring your palm into contact with the wall, and spin your palm counterclockwise, pointing your fingers down toward the floor.
3. Press your palm into the wall by shifting your weight toward your arm.
4. Press your elbow up and open to the ceiling as you press your palm against the wall.
5. Hold for 15 to 20 seconds, and repeat on the opposite arm.
6. Perform three sets.

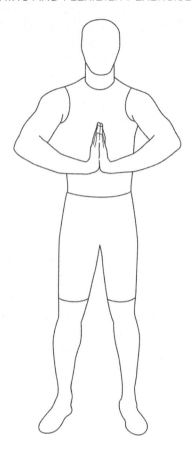

PRAYER HANDS

AFFECTED AREAS

Forearms: flexors, pronators, extensors

Wrists

GOOD FOR:

Achieving the symmetry of this pose calls for you to focus on the midline of your body as you press your hands together and open the front of your chest. Prayer hands may help alleviate pain associated with ailments such as tennis elbow and arthritis.

When you're ready, advance to this dynamic variation. As you stretch through your arms, slowly extend your prayer hands above your head, keeping your palms pressed together, and slowly lower your hands back down toward the center of your chest. Repeat for up to 60 seconds.

To achieve the ultimate symmetry of this stretch, be sure to form a straight line from elbow to elbow and along your forearms while keeping your palms pressed together.

TYPE: STATIC, ACTIVE

INSTRUCTIONS

1. Begin in a comfortable position either standing or sitting.
2. Inhale and press your palms together in front of your chest, with your fingers touching your chin.
3. Exhale as you press the base of your palms, fingers, and thumbs firmly together and lower your hands toward your waist.
4. Hold for 15 to 30 seconds, and repeat three times.

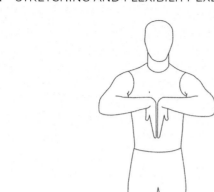

PRAYER HANDS FLEXION

AFFECTED AREAS

Forearms: flexors, pronators, extensors

GOOD FOR:

Your wrists are each made up of eight small bones. Connecting into your wrists and hands are multiple muscles and tendons of your forearms that help control your hand movements. This flexing stretch is wonderful for loosening up the muscles in your forearms, wrists, and hands.

For an added challenge, try moving your hands and fingers from left to right while pressing the tops of your hands together.

You need not try right away to reach a full range of wrist movement in this stretch. Trust your limits and work within them; eventually, a wider range will come to you through practice.

. . .

TYPE: STATIC, ACTIVE
INSTRUCTIONS

1. Begin in a comfortable position either standing or sitting.
2. Inhale and press the tops of your hands together in front of your chest into an inverted Prayer Hands position.
3. Exhale as you focus on keeping contact between the tops of your hands and fingers and lowering your shoulders and elbows.
4. Hold for 10 to 15 seconds.

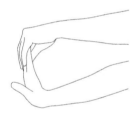

FINGER STRETCH

AFFECTED AREAS
Forearms: flexors, pronators, wrist extensors, hands, and fingers

GOOD FOR:
Hours of scrolling on your computer or texting on your phone can lead to overuse of your fingers, causing stiffness, tenderness, and pain in your arms, elbows, and wrists. Take some time to open up the spaces between your fingers with this simple stretch.

For an added stretch through your wrists, flip your hands over so that your palms are facing up. Now, curl your fingers into tight fists and hold for 10 seconds. Then slowly release your fists and open your hands. Wiggle your fingers and repeat three times.

Your thumbs can easily become more immobile than your fingers, so pay attention to how you splay your hands open. Give extra attention to your thumbs, pulling them gently open and in toward each other.

TYPE: DYNAMIC

INSTRUCTIONS

1. Choose a comfortable place where you can stand easily or can sit with support from a chair.
2. Extend your arms out in front of your chest, keeping your elbows slightly bent.
3. Press your fingers and thumbs together so that there's no space between them, and hold for five seconds.
4. Next, spread your fingers wide open, creating a lot of space between them. Hold for five seconds.
5. Repeat five times.

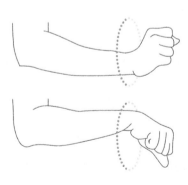

FIST ROTATION

AFFECTED AREAS

Forearms: flexors, pronators, extensors

Neck

GOOD FOR:

Try these deceivingly simple fist rotations at your own leisure. You may discover that your range of motion differs between hands. Enjoy some relief through your neck and arms as an important reminder of the interconnectedness that exists throughout your body.

For a more intense stretch through your wrists and fore-arms, hold a small weighted ball in each hand and wrap your fingers evenly around them. Perform your wrist circles in each direction.

The focus of this exercise is to independently isolate the movement of your wrists from the movement of your fore-arms. Pay attention to when you want to move your forearms and when you are able to fully isolate your wrists: This will reveal where your hands are tightest.

TYPE: STATIC, ACTIVE

INSTRUCTIONS

1. Loosely extend your arms out in front of your body.
2. Turn your palms down, and curl in your fingers to make soft fists.
3. Slowly begin to make isolated circular movements with your fists, keeping your forearms steady.
4. Perform five rotations in one direction, then reverse the direction for another five rotations.
5. Do three sets on each wrist.

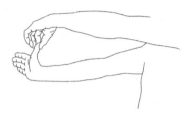

THUMB STRETCH

AFFECTED AREAS

Thumbs: flexors, extensors, pro nadirs

GOOD FOR:

Our hands get a workout all day long: We text, type, play musical instruments, and do various chores. Yet rarely do we take the time to pamper our tired hands and, in particular, our thumbs. These isolated stretches are most impactful when you're fully relaxed.

Turn this stretch into a dynamic exercise and rotate your thumb in circles with your opposite hand. Keep your palm steady as you move your thumb.

ON THE FLY

This is a very soothing stretch that can be done seated, lying down, or standing. It is especially valuable because you can perform it anywhere you go.

TYPE: STATIC, PASSIVE

INSTRUCTIONS

1. Find a comfortable place to sit.
2. Hold your right hand in front of your chest, with your palm facing your chest.
3. Wrap your left hand around your right thumb. Keeping your right hand in line with your forearm, push your thumb downward, and hold for 10 seconds.
4. Flex your wrist toward your chest. Push your thumb toward your forearm, and hold for 10 seconds.
5. Next, extend your wrist so your palm is perpendicular to your chest. Again push on your thumb, and hold for 10 seconds.
6. Repeat on the opposite hand.

FIVE

CHAPTER 5 CHEST AND STOMACH

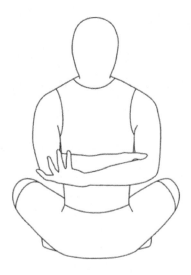

BEHIND-THE-BACK ELBOW-TO-ELBOW GRIP

G **OOD FOR:** This stretch, done properly, allows you to open your chest and shoulder muscles, as well as engage your triceps.

• • •

INSTRUCTIONS:

1. Standing or sitting, exhale as you swing your arms behind you in an arc.
2. Lock your arms and hold, squeezing your arms together.
3. Try to push your chest out.
4. Now, bring your arms back in front of you and repeat the movement once more.

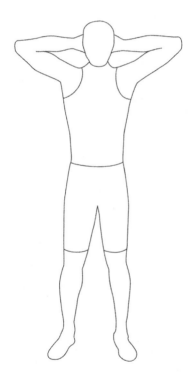

ABOVE-THE-HEAD CHEST STRETCH

GOOD FOR: This stretch opens your chest and stretches your arms and shoulders.

INSTRUCTIONS

1. Standing or sitting, extend your arms above your head on either side of a doorframe (or stable piece of furniture) with your fingers interlocked.
2. Exhale as you lean back into the stretch and hold for one minute.

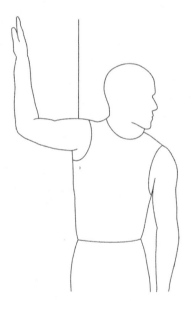

BENT-ARM WALL STRETCH

GOOD FOR: This stretch opens your chest and breathing muscles and helps to keep your spine in a good alignment.

. . .

INSTRUCTIONS:

1. Sitting against any stable, vertical wall with legs extended in front of you, tilt your head back so that you look straight up at the top of the wall.
2. Now rotate your arms backward, creating a small U-shape from shoulder to torso. Hold this position for 10 seconds before repeating on the other side.

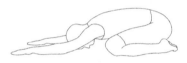

CHILD'S POSE

GOOD FOR: Stretching spine, thighs, hips, and ankles.

INSTRUCTIONS:

1. Get down on all fours, so that your knees are perfectly aligned with your upper leg, and your hands are perfectly aligned with your shoulders.
2. Place the roof of your feet down flat and spread out your knees side to the sides but without moving your feet.
3. Begin to move only your upper body towards the ground.
4. Place your forehead against the ground.
5. Stay on the ground for about 20 seconds and then move up slowly to then go down again.
6. Repeat this motion as many times as you want.

Within stretching and yoga circles, this stretching pose is one of the best out there. It is beginner-friendly, but I recommend doing it as an intermediate. It both stretches and engages multiple muscle groups in your whole body. Likewise, moving up and down gently works out your muscles to create a balanced toned look to your whole body. Get ready for that beach body!

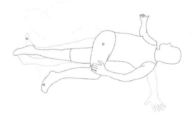

SIDE-LYING PARALLEL ARM CHEST STRETCH

GOOD FOR: This stretch is about aligning your body so that you can free up the chest.

. . .

INSTRUCTIONS:

1. While lying on your side, place your arm on top of your body with a slight bend at the elbow.
2. Push your arm down using the weight of your body, while breathing deep.
3. Feel the stretch through to the shoulder on top and into the shoulder underneath.
4. Repeat this movement 5 times on each side.
5. Gently and slowly stand up to go back to your original position.
6. Repeat this motion 5 times on each side.

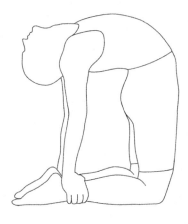

CAMEL POSE

GOOD FOR: Improving posture and counteracting the effects of long-term sitting.

INSTRUCTIONS:

1. Start on your knees, while being upright, having a nice long back and neck.
2. Pick a leg – let's say the right one, as in the illustration above – and move it out in front of you, while your back left foot moves back to stretch your toes against the sturdy ground.
3. Move your out-stretched arms upwards, reaching for the sky.
4. Then meet your left hand with your left heel, leaning your whole upper body backward, creating a nice arch.
5. Help this stretch out with your right arm stretching yourself downward as well
6. Hold for at least 10 seconds and do the same again, but this time switch out your legs and arms.

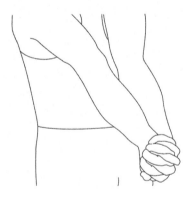

HANDS BEHIND BACK

GOOD FOR: This stretch completely loosens the chest.

• • •

This chest stretch is both simple to execute and very effective. Your chest will feel the stretch, but so will your back!

INSTRUCTIONS:

1. Standing up straight and tall, extend both of your arms behind your back.
2. Take one hand over the other, palms facing outwards.
3. Walk your hands down until you feel a stretch through your shoulders and chest.
4. Repeat these steps up to 5 times.

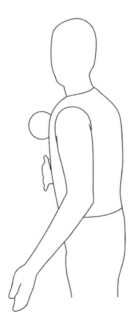

PEC RELEASE

GOOD FOR: Loosening the chest muscles.

This is a great chest stretch for individuals who sit at a desk all day. In addition, it can also help to improve posture.

INSTRUCTIONS:

1. Stand up tall with your feet hip-width apart, and your knees loose.
2. Bend your upper body forward at a 90-degree angle.
3. Drop your chest so that it rests on the top of your thighs, breathe deeply to release tension.
4. Let your arms lie down by your sides while you stretch.
5. Hold this position for at least 20 seconds and then stand up to resume your starting position.

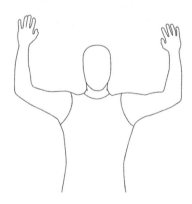

WALL ANGELS

GOOD FOR: Activating the upper back postural muscles that keep your shoulders pushed back.

This stretch is also known as the "V" to "W" stretch .

INSTRUCTIONS:

1. Stand up straight and tall.
2. Shift your weight from your back leg to the front.
3. Move your hands out as you see in the image. Try to push your shoulders in as you move your hands backward,
4. Make sure to hold the stretch for at least 20 seconds.
5. Repeat 3-5 times on each side.

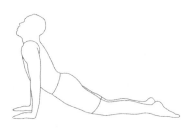

COBRA POSE ABDOMINAL STRETCH

GOOD FOR: This stretch is good for a lot of things like reducing inflammation, and improving sleep, and posture.

Lie face down on the floor with your thumbs directly under the shoulders, legs extended with the tops of your feet on the floor.

•   •   •

INSTRUCTIONS:

1. Tighten your pelvic floor, and tuck your hips downward as you squeeze your glutes.
2. Press the shoulders down and away from your ears.
3. Push through your thumbs and index your fingers as you raise your chest towards the wall in front of you.
4. Relax and repeat.
5. Do 5 repetitions total.

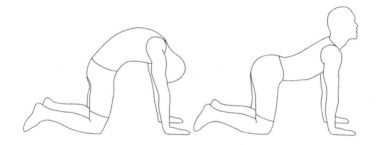

CAT COW POSE STRETCH

GOOD FOR: Strengthens and stretches the spine and neck.

INSTRUCTIONS:

1. Begin by kneeling on all four with your hands in the line below your shoulders and your hips in line with your knees. Lengthen your neck and roll your shoulders back.
2. Inhale and scoop your abdomen toward the floor, arching your back, and gaze forward.
3. As you exhale, tuck in your abdomen and slowly curl your back toward the ceiling while tucking in your chin toward your chest. Think of forming an upside-down U with your body.
4. Hold for a moment and inhale as you return to the neutral position.
5. Repeat 10 to 15 times.

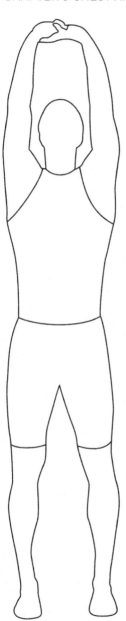

STANDING AB STRETCH

GOOD FOR: Loosening all the abs and releasing tension in stomach.

INSTRUCTIONS:

1. Stand up tall and straight with your feet shoulder-width apart.
2. Place your hands in front of your chest, palms facing outward.
3. As you inhale, draw your arms back and away from the body so you are stretching the arms out in front of you, while keeping a slight bend in the elbows.
4. As you exhale, dip down to rest the forehead on your upper arms.
5. Hold this position for at least 15-20 seconds.
6. Repeat this motion 5 times.

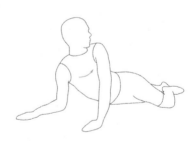

OBLIQUE STRETCH

"The Kneeling Oblique Stretch"

GOOD FOR: adding extra support to the back muscles and prevent back pain and injury.

INSTRUCTIONS:

1. Start on all fours, try to stack your knees directly underneath your buttocks in a straight line.
2. Orient your feet so your toes are touching the ground.
3. Then go down onto your elbows still lying flat on the ground, resting your head in your palms.
4. At all times try to have a straight back.
5. Try to hold this for at least 1 minute, or longer.

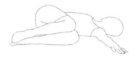

TWISTING CROCODILE STRETCH

This pose is great if you have a desk job, as it stretches and lengthens your spine.

GOOD FOR: Loosening tension in the back. The deeper the stretch the more the tension in the back is released.

INSTRUCTIONS:

1. Stand up straight and tall with your feet hip-width apart, knees soft.
2. Rotate the torso and hips to the left in one fluid motion, with arms extended at shoulder level.
3. Let the left arm remain extended straight to the side while turning the head to look over the left shoulder.
4. Return to the starting position.
5. Repeat the movement on the other side.

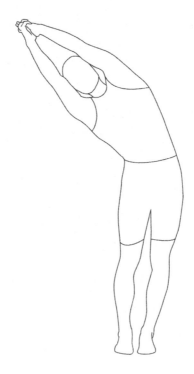

STANDING SIDE BEND

This stretch helps to elongate your spine, especially if you have a desk job.

GOOD FOR: Improves spinal mobility, and breathing efficiency.

INSTRUCTIONS:

1. Stand up straight and tall with your feet shoulder-width apart, knees soft.
2. Bend sideways to the right, keeping your hips and back in line.
3. To make sure you are maintaining the same angle of the bend as when you first began, check that your torso is still vertical while bent at 90 degrees.
4. Repeat on the other side.

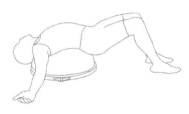

EXERCISE BALL AB STRETCH

This stretch helps to open up your hips, which will help you if you spend a lot of time sitting.

GOOD FOR: Releases tension in the chest, back, and tailbone.

· · ·

INSTRUCTIONS:

1. Place an exercise ball behind your back.
2. Sit down on the ball until you feel a gentle pull in your lower abs.
3. Bend forward at 90 degrees, keeping the back straight and chest lifted.
4. Hold this pose for at least 20 seconds, breathing deep.
5. Repeat 5 times.

SIX

LEGS & GLUTES

Your legs are the foundation of your body, supplying support and stability. Toned, flexible muscles in your thighs, knees, calves, ankles and feet can minimize aches and pains. Your legs also help to improve posture, help prevent injuries, and speed recovery time after engaging in sports or workouts.

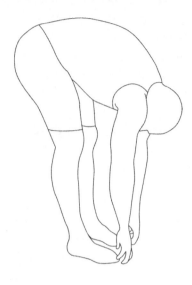

TOE TOUCH STANDING

AFFECTED AREAS

Thighs: hamstrings

Calves

Buttocks: glutes

GOOD FOR:

Moving through this Toe Touch stretch is a great way to feel the connection of muscles from your hips, along the backs of your legs, and down to your feet. The inversion also helps get your blood flowing.

Hold a weighted ball in your hands to begin. As you bend forward, lower the ball toward your toes, allowing gravity to deepen the stretch along the backs of your legs.

ON THE FLY:

This stretch is great for any time you feel tightness in the back of your legs. Find a comfortable location that allows you enough space to reach for your toes, and go for it.

· · ·

INSTRUCTIONS:

1. Stand up straight, lengthening your spine, and place your feet shoulder-width apart.
2. Lower your head and slowly curl your torso forward, one vertebra at a time, bending from your hips. Allow your arms to dangle loosely beneath you.
3. If you can, touch your toes, and breathe deeply, inhaling and exhaling.
4. Hold for 10 seconds.
5. Roll up slowly through your lower back and spine, and return to a neutral position.
6. Repeat three to five times.

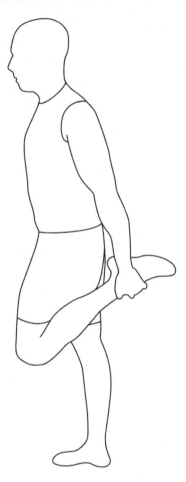

STANDING QUADRICEP STRETCH

AFFECTED AREAS

Thighs: quadriceps

Shins: tibialis

GOOD FOR:

If you've ever been sitting for so long that when you stand up that the front of your hips feel stuck and cramped, this stretch may be beneficial for you. Release tension and stiffness from sedentary postures with this standing quadricep stretch.

For a stretch along your outer thigh and iliotibial band, grab your raised foot with the opposite hand. Allow your raised leg to turn out slightly, and bring your heel across to the opposite hip.

Press your pelvis forward, and keep your hips flat to the front without arching your lower spine. If needed, use a wall or a chair for balance.

INSTRUCTIONS:

1. Stand straight with your feet together and engage your abs.
2. Bend your left knee, bringing your left foot up behind you.
3. Reach your left arm behind you, and wrap your hand around the top of your left foot. Bring your right hand onto your right hip to help with balance or let it hang at your side.
4. Pull your left heel in toward your left hip and hold for 10 to 15 seconds.
5. Return to a neutral position, and repeat two to three times on each leg.

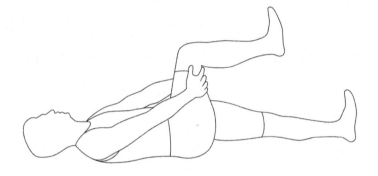

BENT- KNEE HAMSTRING STRETCH

AFFECTED AREAS

Thighs: hamstrings, quadriceps

Calves:

GOOD FOR:

Utilizing the pull of gravity to stretch your leg makes this simple Hamstring Stretch great for all ages and body types. This move is good for warming up before a workout, cooling down after a run, or searching for relief from lower back pain.

Use a resistance band or rolled-up towel to maximize your range in this stretch. Wrap the band under your raised foot, and hold the ends with both hands. As you straighten your leg, use the band to pull your leg in closer toward your chest.

If you have very tight hamstrings, it may cause you to hike up your shoulders and tense the surrounding neck muscles. Press the back of your neck flat against the floor and gently press your shoulders down away from your ears.

INSTRUCTIONS:

1. Lie on your back with your knees bent. Place both feet flat on the floor.
2. Lift your left leg into the air, and wrap your hands behind your leg just above your knee.
3. Engage your abs, flex your left foot, and slowly straighten your knee.
4. Hold here for 15 to 20 seconds, and return to a neutral position.
5. Repeat three to five times on each leg.

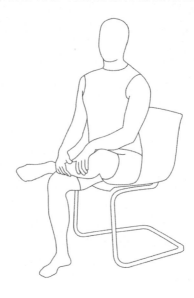

PIRIFORMIS STRETCH

AFFECTED AREAS

Shins:

Feet:

Toes

GOOD FOR:

Many of us spend hours on our feet daily and don't give them enough attention. Pain in your hips, knees, and lower back is sometimes related to how you stand on your feet. Try this isolated Foot Sickle stretch to rejuvenate your outer shins and ankles.

To get a deeper stretch through your ankle joint, hold your foot just below your toes. Pull the middle of your foot up toward you while keeping the support of the other hand on your shin.

This stretch can be done either seated in a chair or with the support of the floor. You can do this stretch anywhere, just remember to take off your shoes first so you can isolate the stretch accordingly.

INSTRUCTIONS:

1. Find a comfortable seated position, and bring your right foot up to cross over your left knee.
2. Support your right shin with your right hand while you wrap your left hand around your right toes.
3. Isolate your toes and your right foot, then pull your right toes toward your left shoulder.
4. Hold for 10 to 15 seconds and repeat on the opposite foot.
5. Perform three sets.

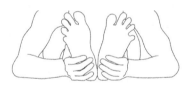

TOE STRETCH

AFFECTED AREAS
Feet: extensors
Arches of feet:
Toes
GOOD FOR:

Your range of motion may vary significantly from toe to toe as you try out these easy Toe Stretch isolations. In addition to targeting your toes, this stretch series soothes tired ankles and arches. It's perfect for general foot pain and for cooling down overworked feet.

When stretching your toes, try moving them in a new

direction. Instead of tugging them apart, push them up and down, working each neighboring toe against the other.

Even though your toes are small, they play an important part in carrying and dispersing the weight of your body. to care for them and be gentle when stretching.

INSTRUCTIONS:

1. Find a comfortable seated position, and cross your right ankle over your left knee.
2. Begin by pulling your big toe away from your second toe.
3. Next, tug apart your second toe and middle toes.
4. Continue separating your toes this way down to your pinky toe.
5. Breathe deeply as you stretch, and repeat three to five times on each foot.

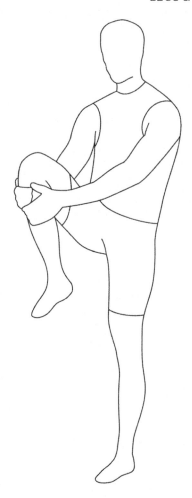

HIGH KNEE WALKING

AFFECTED AREAS

Thighs: quadriceps, hamstrings

Buttocks: glutes

GOOD FOR:

This high knee stretch has many benefits. Not only are you stretching through your knees and upper legs, but you're also improving strength, coordination, and circulation in your core, exterior leg muscles, and hip joints. This dynamic stretch is ideal for warming up before a run.

For an added challenge, strap on some light ankle weights and proceed slowly. This will serve to strengthen your quadriceps as well as improve your balance. Perform five repetitions on each leg.

This is a simple exercise that you can do anywhere. It is especially useful as a warm-up before various sports and aerobic workouts. Engage your core to help you keep the movement fluid and controlled.

INSTRUCTIONS:

1. Begin by standing straight with your feet hip-width apart. Place your hands on your hips.
2. Shift your weight onto your left foot, engage your core, and bring your left knee up high so that your hamstrings are parallel to the floor.
3. Lower your foot to the floor, step forward, and repeat with the opposite leg.
4. Continue walking for 10 repetitions on each leg.
5. Turn around and repeat three times.

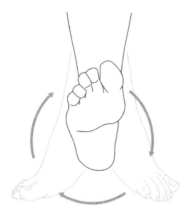

ANKLE CIRCLES

AFFECTED AREAS

Shins:

Arches of feet:

Toes

GOOD FOR:

When you move your body parts in a circular manner, you help promote circulation, mobility, and relaxation. Here, by isolating your ankle joint and moving it in a smooth circular motion through its maximum range, you can relax your tired, achy feet and enhance their flexibility.

Increase the range of motion by using your hand to assist your ankle through a wider circle. Place your left leg on your right thigh, and press your right palm against the sole of your left foot. Hold the sides of your arch and gently rotate your ankle in each direction.

This stretch can be done just about anywhere, with or without your shoes on. If your feet are feeling achy or swollen, find a wall to help with your balance and circle your ankles a few times in each direction.

. . .

INSTRUCTIONS:

1. Stand straight with your feet hip-width apart, and place your hands on your hips.
2. Bend your right knee, and lift your right foot from the floor.
3. Trace a small circle counterclockwise with your right foot by pointing your toes down to the floor, out to your right, up to the ceiling, and in toward your left leg.
4. Perform five circles, then reverse the direction, tracing a circle clockwise.
5. Repeat five times on each foot.

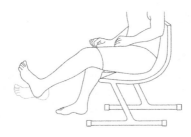

POINTE & FLEX

AFFECTED AREAS
    Shins
    Calves
    Arches of feet
    Toes
    GOOD FOR:
Unless you are a ballerina and are always on your toes, your feet are probably in a flexed position most of the day. Try

this stretch to invigorate tired feet and loosen up the tightness in the joints of your lower leg.

For an inversion, wrap a resistance band or rolled-up towel behind the soles of your feet. Pull firmly on the band as you flex your feet. Push the backs of your legs into the floor, and push away with your heels as you curl your toes back toward your shins.

When you're able to take a break from your daily routine, find a quiet location to sit either on the floor or in a chair, slip off your shoes, and work your feet through this pointe stretch.

INSTRUCTIONS:

1. Sit comfortably and extend your legs straight in front of you.
2. Curl your feet and toes away from your shins and toward the floor, bringing each foot into a full pointe.
3. Hold for 15 seconds and return to a neutral position.
4. Now flex your feet by engaging your calves and pushing out through your heels while pulling your toes back toward you.
5. Hold for 10 seconds and return to neutral.
6. Repeat three to five times.

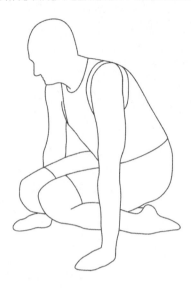

TIBIALIS KNEE STRETCH

AFFECTED AREAS

Shins:

Calves:

GOOD FOR:

Utilizing the force of gravity, this move allows you to shoot down through your hips and lengthen your shins, calves, and feet. This restorative stretch relieves stiffness through your legs and feet. It may also help decrease calf and ankle swelling after air travel.

When you're ready for a much more advanced version of this stretch, try the yoga-based Reclining Hero Pose. Kneel with your feet wider than hip-width apart, and place your arms behind you. Slowly lower your back toward the floor.

If you have knee pain and are not able to kneel comfortably in the basic pose, tuck a folded blanket or towel under your hips for extra support.

. . .

INSTRUCTIONS:

1. Begin by kneeling on all fours on a solid surface with the tops of your feet on the floor.
2. Slowly bring your legs together so that they touch.
3. Gradually tip your hips back toward your feet and come into a full kneel, bringing your hips to your heels.
4. Engage your abs and sit up straight. Rest your hands on your thighs and breathe deeply.
5. Hold for 30 seconds and repeat three times.

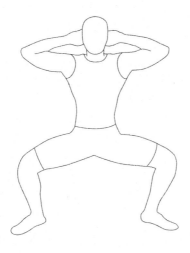

SUMO SQUAT

AFFECTED AREAS

Thighs: quadriceps, hamstrings, abductors, adductors
GOOD FOR:

Take a wide-open stance and come into the Sumo stretch to activate and lengthen muscles deep in your hips and legs. You'll also build stamina and strength through your core.

Holding the correct sumo position is challenging—you need to bend your knees deeply all while keeping your abs in and up. This is a great stretch to do before working out, running, or playing sports.

Challenge the strength in your core and in your legs by holding a weighted medicine ball or kettlebell overhead as you bend your knees and slowly lower into your sumo position.

This move can be performed anywhere, assuming your clothing allows for it. Find a space wide enough for your squat position and be sure to keep your core and back muscles engaged the whole time.

INSTRUCTIONS:

1. Stand with your feet about three to four feet apart.
2. Engage your core and bend your knees, bringing your hips into a squat position with your knees in line over your ankles and your hamstrings parallel to the floor.
3. Rest your hands on your knees.
4. Hold here for 20 to 30 seconds and return to a neutral position.
5. Repeat three times.

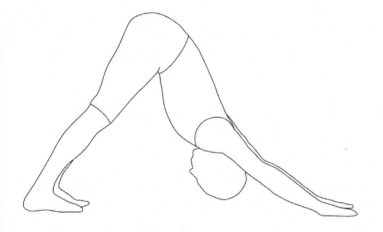

DOWNWARD DOG

AFFECTED AREAS

Buttocks: glutes

Thighs: adductors, abductors, hamstrings

Calves:

Shoulders: deltoids

GOOD FOR:

The Downward Dog is a classic, energizing yoga pose. No matter your background or age, this stretch maximizes length and strength through your entire body as you push against the floor with your arms and legs. You'll also really get your blood flowing.

For a challenge, lift your heels off the floor and come to balance on the balls of your feet. Take a slight bend in your knees, and push your hips up high and back behind you.

The more firmly you push down into your heels and feet, the deeper of a stretch you will feel through your lower body and back.

INSTRUCTIONS:

1. Kneel on all fours on a firm flat surface with your hands in line with your shoulders and your knees, directly below your hips.
2. Splay your fingers open, and push down into your hands and heels. Inhale deeply to prepare.
3. On exhale, lift your knees from the floor, straighten your legs, and raise your hips toward the ceiling. Think of creating a triangle shape with your body.
4. Engage your core, and lengthen your spine as you focus your gaze on your abs.
5. Hold here for 30 to 45 seconds and return to a neutral position. Repeat twice.

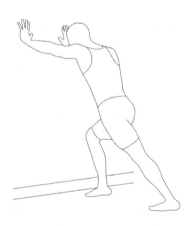

WALL-ASSISTED CALF STRETCH

AFFECTED AREAS

Calves

Shins

Thighs: hamstrings

GOOD FOR:

This intense stretch for your calves and Achilles tendons is a very familiar stretch that's especially popular with runners. With the support of a wall, you can push deeper into your lower leg while maintaining your balance the entire time.

Once you've found your comfort zone in the basic calf stretch, intensify the movement by turning your feet. As you stretch your right calf, shift your toes slightly outward to the right, then to the left. You'll feel the stretch along the sides of your calf.

This is a stretch that should be done gently, with little force. Take care not to overstretch your calf muscles or Achilles tendon: Press your heel down slowly each time.

INSTRUCTIONS:

1. Stand straight facing a wall or another solid surface.
2. Place your hands on the wall at shoulder height to support your weight.
3. Bend your left knee, and step your right foot back about two to three feet behind you.
4. Straighten your right knee, and press your right heel down as you gently bend your left knee deeper.
5. Hold here for 20 to 30 seconds, return to a neutral position, and repeat on the opposite leg.
6. Perform three repetitions.

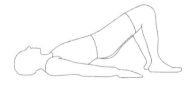

GLUTE BRIDGES

AFFECTED AREAS
  Glutes
  Groin
  Thighs: hamstrings
  GOOD FOR:

This simple stretch is amazing for people that have very long days at work. Sometimes those days can lead to back pain and body aches. Use this stretch to help alleviate that pain while strengthening your lower body. This stretch will also work your abs.

TYPE: STATIC, PASSIVE
  INSTRUCTIONS:

1. Lie face up on the floor, with your knees bent and feet flat on the ground. Keep your arms at your side with your palms down.
2. Lift your hips off the ground until your knees, hips, and shoulders form a straight line.
3. Squeeze your glutes hard and keep your abs tight so you don't overextend your back during the exercise.
4. Hold the bridged position for 3-5 seconds before easing back down.
5. Start with one set of 10 and then continue to two sets of 10 as your body gets stronger.

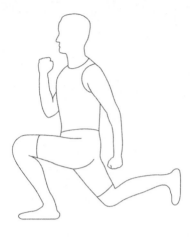

FORWARD LUNGE

AFFECTED AREAS

Thighs: hamstrings, quadriceps, adductors

Buttocks: glutes

Shins:

GOOD FOR:

The Forward Lunge reaches deep into your hips and opens the muscles around the front and the back of your legs and pelvis. Because you need to bend deeply through your hips, be sure to thoroughly warm up your back, hips, and legs before you attempt this exercise.

Intensify the stretch by holding the lowered position for 10 to 15 seconds.

Protect your knee joints by making sure that you do not overextend your front knee. As you lunge forward, your knee should not extend any further forward than your ankle.

INSTRUCTIONS:

1. Begin by standing straight with your feet hip-width apart. Place your hands on your hips.
2. Step your right foot far forward, pressing down with your heel first.
3. Shift your weight over your right leg, and lower your right knee toward the floor.
4. Press your right heel into the floor to push you back to the neutral position.
5. Repeat on the opposite leg, and perform five times per side.

SEVEN
NECK AND BACK

Whether you are old, middle-aged, or in your 20s, we all have experienced back and neck pain from a long day of work. Especially in this age of cell phones, our necks are constantly bent. These stretches help to loosen the muscles in the neck and also help you to maintain amazing posture. All while relieving those aches and pains in the neck and back.

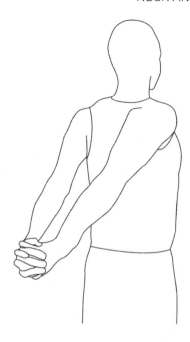

SEATED SHOULDER SQUEEZE

Affected Areas: Shoulders, Arms, Lower Back.

GOOD FOR: Shoulder and upper limb stability:

INSTRUCTIONS:

This stretch is excellent for reducing stress and also lowering some of the tension in our lower back from a long day at work.

1. Sit on the floor, or anywhere with space, with your knees bent and feet flat on the floor.
2. Interlock your hands together behind your lower back.
3. Straighten and extend your arms and squeeze your shoulder blades together.
4. Do this for 3-5 seconds, and then release.
5. You want to do this anywhere from 5 to 10 times.

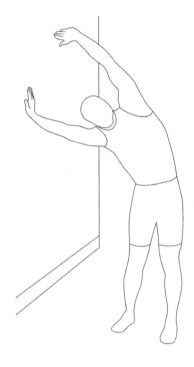

WALL-ASSISTED SIDE BEND

AFFECTED AREAS
  Back:

Abdomen: abdominal obliques

Many of us favor one side of our body and build tightness around overused muscles. This deep side bend lengthens the muscles in the middle of your back, one side at a time, so you can target the areas that need more flexibility.

Intensify the stretch by placing your hands higher on the doorframe. You'll engage more muscles all through the side of your body and along your spine.

This side bend is a very effective, deep stretch that you can perform anywhere you find a door.

GOOD FOR: lengthen the abdominal, hip, and thigh muscles.

INSTRUCTIONS:

1. Stand straight with your feet together and about an arm's distance to the left of a doorframe.
2. Keeping your body facing forward, grab the edge of the door frame with both hands, left over right, at about shoulder height.
3. Lean away from the doorframe, shifting your hips toward your left.
4. Hold for 30 seconds and repeat three times per side.

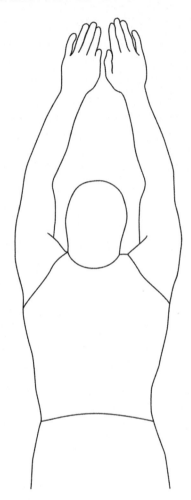

WALL-ASSISTED UPPER-BACK STRETCH

AFFECTED AREAS

Upper back:

Neck:

Poor posture and slouching can often lead to upper back pain, as can prolonged hours sitting at a desk or driving a car.

This simple stretch targets the muscles in your upper and middle back, lengthening the muscles along your spine and releasing pressure between your shoulder blades.

Engage additional muscles along the sides of your neck by turning your head slowly to your right and holding for five seconds. Repeat to the opposite side.

GOOD FOR: Undoing the effects of bad posture.

INSTRUCTIONS:

1. Stand facing a wall with your feet hip-width apart.
2. Press your palms into the wall at shoulder height.
3. Step about two feet away from the wall.
4. Turn your gaze down at your feet and pull your shoulders away from the wall while pressing your hands firmly into the wall.
5. Hold for 30 seconds and repeat three to four times.

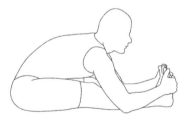

SEATED FORWARD BEND

AFFECTED AREAS
    Upper back:
    Neck:

Although it's not quite an inversion, by bowing your head in this stretch, you can feel that it really gets your blood flowing. This gentle stretch also soothes tightness in your upper back and is a good exercise for relieving daily stress.

Clasp your hands behind your back, rounding your shoulders, and perform the exercise as above. You'll feel a slightly deeper stretch in your upper back.

GOOD FOR: calming your mind and relieving stress, this pose stretches your spine, shoulders, and hamstrings. It also stimulates the liver, kidneys, ovaries, and uterus—and can help improve digestion.

INSTRUCTIONS:

1. Sit down and put your feet in front of you together.
2. Slowly bend forward from your hips and let your hands rest on your calves or as close to your toes as you can.
3. Inhale to prepare. Try to pull your body and your legs close together.
4. As you exhale, tilt your head downward, turning your gaze toward your knees.
5. Hold for a slow exhale, and slowly repeat the movement 10 to 20 times.

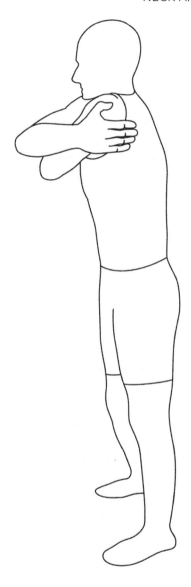

BEAR HUG

AFFECTED AREAS

Upper back:

Shoulders:

Nothing like a bear hug to release tension and tight knots between your shoulder blades. This stretch may also alleviate the stiffness associated with bursitis and frozen shoulder.

Perform the Bear Hug as above, except tilt your chin into your chest and hold for 20 seconds. This extra movement will further lengthen the muscles running along your upper back.

GOOD FOR: helps to alleviate discomfort in the shoulder blades.

INSTRUCTIONS:

1. Stand straight in a comfortable stance.
2. Cross your arms in front of your chest, reaching your hands around your back and placing them on the opposite shoulder blade.
3. Press your hands into your shoulder blades and lift your elbows to shoulder height.
4. Pull your shoulders away from your body and hold for 20 to 30 seconds.
5. Release and cross your arms with the opposite arm on top and repeat twice per side.

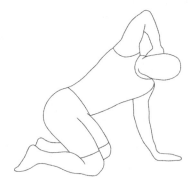

QUADRUPED ROTATIONS

AFFECTED AREAS

Upper and middle back:

Abdomen: abdominal obliques

Whenever you make a twisting motion in your torso, you're relying on the mobility of your thoracic spine in your upper and middle back. By targeting your T spine, this stretch helps to increase your range of motion in your daily activities —whether you're just reaching across a table, throwing a ball, or dancing the samba.

Perform the exercise as above, except as you raise your arm, and sit back on your heels. This extra movement lengthens your spine as you rotate.

GOOD FOR: This stretch is perfect for increasing T-Spine mobility without much lower back movement.

INSTRUCTIONS:

1. Begin kneeling on all fours with your hands in line with your shoulders and your knees in line with your hips.
2. Place your left hand behind your head and lift your elbow out to your side.
3. Inhale as you rotate through your thoracic spine and reach your left elbow down toward the floor, keeping your neck aligned with your spine and your hips stable.
4. As you exhale, slowly twist your torso up, readying your elbow toward the ceiling.
5. Perform this movement 10 times, and repeat three times on each side.

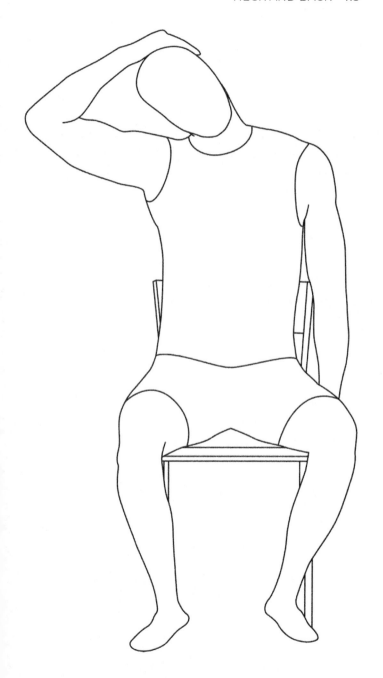

SEATED NECK STRETCH

AFFECTED AREAS: Neck

Most people will stretch out their entire bodies but will forget to stretch their necks. It is extremely important to strengthen the muscles in your neck in today's day and age. Especially since we spend almost all of our time looking at our phones, forcing our necks to be in awkward positions for hours on hours a day.

GOOD FOR: This stretch is perfect for a work day. It helps to release tension in the neck from looking at that computer and typing the whole day.

INSTRUCTIONS:

1. Stand with feet shoulder-width apart, or you can do this stretch sitting down with your back straight and chest lifted.
2. Place your left hand on the right side of your right ear and gently pull down, stretching the neck.
3. Do this on both sides.
4. Hold for 30 seconds to 2 minutes.

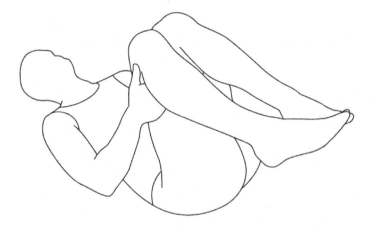

DOUBLE KNEE TO CHEST

AFFECTED AREAS

Lower back:

Buttocks: glutes

The Double Knee to Chest stretch is one of the gentlest yet most effective spinal decompression exercises you can do. As you curl your legs into your chest and roll your back down, you'll feel a soothing massage along your spinal column. This stretch works wonders for lower back pain.

Try this rolling motion for a gentle spinal massage. Clasp your hands together behind your knees and slowly roll forward lifting one vertebra at a time off the floor. Gently roll back down.

GOOD FOR: This stretch helps to relieve pressure along the entire spinal nerves.

INSTRUCTIONS:

1. Lie on the floor with your knees bent.
2. Bring one leg at a time into your chest and wrap your hands around your shins just below your knees.
3. Gently pull your knees closer to your chest, and hold for 15 to 20 seconds.
4. Return to the neutral position and repeat three times.

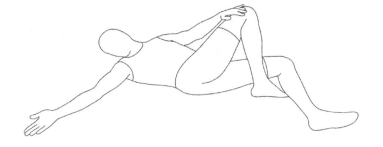

LOWER-BACK ROTATION

AFFECTED AREAS

Lower back:

Abdomen: abdominal obliques

Chronic lower back pain is a major health issue in sedentary societies such as ours. Developing flexibility in your lower back, along your lumbar spine, can minimize pain and improve functional movement. A limber lower back also helps realign your posture and prevent injury.

Intensify the stretch by crossing your legs at your thighs and then dropping your knees to the side. You'll feel it in your lower back as well as your glutes.

Keep your knees pressed together to gain the most benefit from this stretch. If your knees keep separating, place a small rolled-up towel between your knees and squeeze them together.

GOOD FOR: While this is an obvious back stretch that will benefit the back, you may not realize it at first glance, but this stretch is also excellent for a low-intensity ab workout.

INSTRUCTIONS:

1. Lie on your back with your knees bent and your arms extended out to your sides with palms facing up.
2. Press your knees and feet together, and lower your knees to your left side as far as you can go without straining.
3. Keep your shoulders and arms pressed to the floor.
4. Hold for 20 to 30 seconds, return to neutral and repeat on the opposite side.

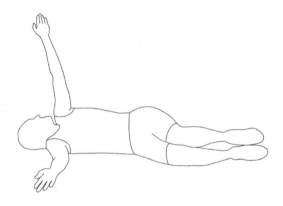

OPEN BOOK STRETCH

AFFECTED AREAS
   Middle back:
   Buttocks:
   Abdomen: external obliques

GOOD FOR: This chest opener helps you regain mobility in your middle back along your thoracic spine. If you tend to slouch and roll your shoulders forward, this stretch can help improve your postural alignment and loosen up the tightness in your T spine.

Add a dynamic movement to this stretch. Lie on your side

with knees bent, and press your left hand on your right thigh. Extend your right hand on the floor in line with your shoulders. Now open your right arm, lifting it straight overhead and over onto the floor on your right while extending your lower leg in line with your body. Hold for a few seconds, return to neutral, and repeat on the opposite side.

INSTRUCTIONS

1. Lie on your right side with your knees bent and legs stacked on top of each other.
2. Start with both arms extended out in front of you.
3. Next, raise your top hand toward the ceiling, and like a clock move one hand to the other.
4. Make sure you keep your legs in one position.
5. For an even better stretch, try to stretch your hands and fingers while doing this stretch.
6. Return to neutral and repeat three times on each side.

EIGHT

CHAPTER 8 ADVANCED STRETCHING

T he following positions are for advanced stretches for men and should not be attempted by a beginner or intermediate without either professional help or oversight.

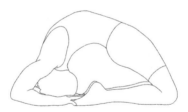

THE KING PIGEON POSE STRETCH

GOOD FOR: This stretch opens the hips and relieves pressures in the muscles we use for everyday walking, running, and exercise. Surprisingly, this is also a really good stretch to raise energy.

. . .

INSTRUCTIONS

1. Begin by sitting on your knees with a straight neck and long back.
2. Once you have your balance, begin to arch your back backward as much as you can until you hit the ground with your palms behind you.
3. Slowly move further down so you are on your elbows, touching the crown of your head on the ground itself.
4. Hold for as long as you can at whatever arch you have managed to get to. Remember, don't overexert yourself.

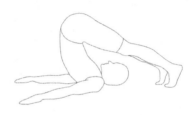

THE ROLLOVER STRETCH

GOOD FOR: An advanced stretch like this will work everything from the top of your back to the heels of your feet. However, you should mostly feel this stretch in your back. Remember, always roll back slowly to avoid damaging your neck.

INSTRUCTIONS:

1. Begin with laying on your back.

2. Keep your arms stretched down your side and palms flat on the ground.
3. Begin to swing your legs up and behind your head.
4. Do this multiple times, it may look silly, but it is incredibly healthy for your body.

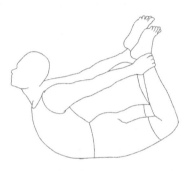

THE BOW STRETCH

GOOD FOR: This stretch opens your shoulders directly from the front of your body. It can help to improve mobility and posture.

INSTRUCTIONS:

1. Start by laying flat on your stomach, enjoying the relaxation.
2. Now start to slowly bend backward, grabbing your feet with your hands. The left-hand grabs your left leg and the right-hand to your right leg.
3. Keep a nice and long neck, looking down into the ground.
4. Begin to create an arch, or a bowl, using your arms, legs, and core.
5. Hold it for a bit, then repeat it.

This pose is very beneficial for your core, and both stretches and tones your body.

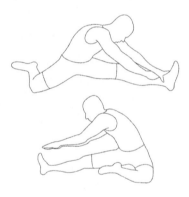

HURDLE STRETCH

GOOD FOR: A stretch like this is amazing for stress relief. It also can be an amazing stretch for starting your day. It may not seem advanced, but this is a stretch that you can hurt your leg muscles with so you want to be sure that you are not over-stretching.

· · ·

INSTRUCTIONS:

1. Start by sitting on the ground with your legs stretched out side-by-side, and with a long back and neck as well.
2. Then pick a side to bend backward, start with your right.
3. Push out your left leg stretched to the left side.
4. And begin now with your arms stretched out to form a bow.
5. Hold here for as long as you can.
6. Repeat with your other leg.

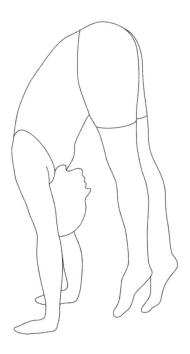

TIP TOE CANNONBALL; TOE AND FOOT STRETCH

GOOD FOR: This is an amazing Tailbone stretch. In addition, you will feel this stretch in your heels and wrists.

INSTRUCTIONS

1. Start by being in a hunched frog position; on both your feet and your hands.
2. Then shift your weight forward, while pressing sideways against your study arms
3. Do this slowly until you are raising your body and you have found your balance point being sturdy on the ground.
4. Stretch your feet behind you and hold for as long as you can.

This exercise is amazing since it betters your balance. It also focuses on neglected areas such as the feet, and you are toning your muscles on your arm as well all in one exercise.

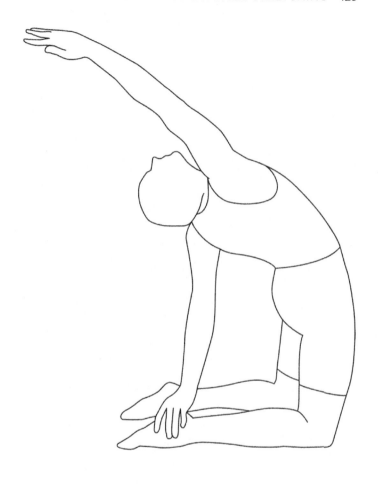

THE HALF CAMEL POSE STRETCH

GOOD FOR: This stretch is good for opening up the arms and shoulders. An additional fact is it helps to stimulate the digestive and respiratory systems!

INSTRUCTIONS:

1. Start on your knees, while being upright, having a nice long back and neck.
2. Start with your right leg and move it out in front of you, while your back left foot moves back to stretch your toes against the sturdy ground.
3. Move your out-stretched arms upwards, reaching for the sky.
4. Then meet your left hand with your left heel, leaning your whole upper body backward, creating a nice arch.
5. Help this stretch out with your right arm stretching yourself downward as well.
6. Hold for at least 10 seconds and do the same again, but this time switch out your legs and arms.

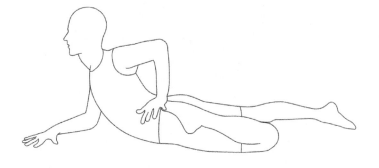

THE HALF FROG POSE STRETCH

GOOD FOR: This is an amazing stretch for runners and cyclists, it opens the body up and is an excellent warm up stretch.

INSTRUCTIONS:

1. Start with being flat on your stomach.
2. Begin now to move your arms underneath your head and lift your upper body upwards.
3. When you have gotten to a nice upward arch, pick an arm, any arm, and bend your leg linked with that arm, for example, see illustration.
4. Try to bend your leg as much as you can, if you hit your upper leg then that is your goal.
5. Stay in this position for at least 15 seconds or more.
6. This position is perfect if you have knee pain or want to work out your lower back and stretch out your hamstring.

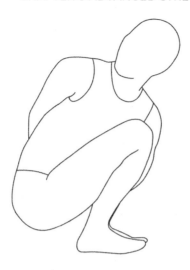

THE NOOSE POSE STRETCH

GOOD FOR: This stretch is good for strengthening the abs, thighs, groin, and abdomen. It is good for relieving asthma, and increases blood circulation in your entire chest area.

INSTRUCTIONS:

1. Start by going down in a squat, not using your arms on the ground but holding yourself up using your feet and bent legs.
2. Then intermingle your hands together in a strong link underneath both your shins.
3. Slowly and being aware of your body, especially your lower back, begin to turn on your core's axis behind you while twisting.
4. Get as much of a twist in as you comfortably can, stay this way for at least 10 seconds.
5. Do this again with the other side.

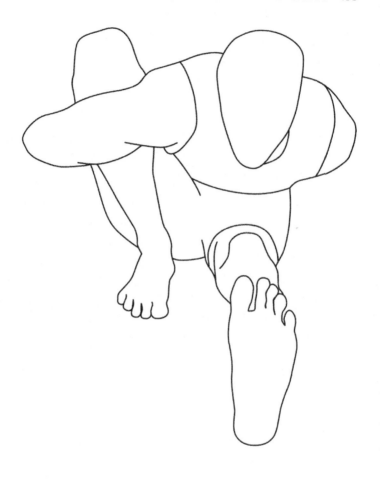

SAGE MARICHI 1 STRETCH

GOOD FOR: This is a good stretch to relieve lower back pain.

INSTRUCTIONS:

1. Begin in a nice straight sitting position with your legs straight out.
2. Pick a leg, any leg, and stretch it out. The other leg should be moved and bent up to your chest.
3. Interlace your arms as much as you can behind your back.
4. Begin to bend your upper body forward towards your stretched-out leg.
5. After you're done with the first leg, switch and perform the stretch with the other.

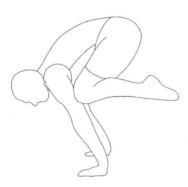

THE CROW POSE STRETCH

This is an advanced position that will take training to perfect. A beginner or even an intermediate shouldn't try this without professional oversight.

GOOD FOR: This stretch is amazing for building strength and balance. The more you do this stretch, you will be surprised to see how much strength you gain.

INSTRUCTIONS:

1. Start by going down in a squat.
2. Then rock your hands and arms gently, moving them slowly more and more.
3. Slowly lift your legs using your core and back strength, while using the tension against your arms from your legs as the stabilization you need for balance.

If you can get this move down, then it will do wonders for you. It will propel your balance to the next level; tone your triceps, and build up your back and core strength.

CONCLUSION

So, you've now learned the benefits of stretching, the reasons why you should stretch, and all of these different exercises. So now you're wondering "Where do I start?". Well, the easiest way to start is to basically just get up and get going. Yes, it is as simple as it sounds. If you have some doubts before beginning, that's normal. It is important to get a basic understanding of our own bodies and how they function. This isn't meant to be an in-depth analysis of the human body, but instead, coming to focus on our bodies, especially as they age. We need to take notice of how our bodies start telling us certain things, so a core idea of how muscles, tendons, and bone structures work is always recommended. Seeing how we, as humans, instinctively perform some sort of stretch during our daily lives, getting into stretch routines is as simple as can be.

Once we understand our bodies, we can actively start to look at area-specific types of exercises/stretches that will benefit those areas the most with the least likelihood of injury.

Keep in mind that it would annoy anyone if they were to experience a lack of motion, body aches and pains, and muscle pains while performing everyday easy-to-handle activities. Now remember that as we age our bodies become more susceptible to the above, and our bodies become frailer. Practicing safe stretching exercises will aid you in many ways, and that is why you should never be intimidated by any exercise in this book. These stretches are all intended to help you and your body to operate at the best version of itself.

It is generally understood that any type of stretching pose, if held correctly, and for the exact recommended time, might start out as being a little tough on our bodies. This is more true for people aged 55 and up, but, as most of us know, even though it starts out not quite as easy as we thought, any act repeated daily and done correctly will, over time, become so easy that the effort we put into it would start to seem like no effort at all.

One thing to keep in mind is that there are no set expectations for anyone who is just starting on their journey into stretching; it isn't expected that you master every possible stretching exercise in one day. Stretching is done at your own pace and at a level with which you are comfortable. Always remember to consult your doctor before attempting any type of strenuous physical activity, ascertaining your level of performance as well as your limitations.

Another thing to remember is that this book is geared towards you, the strong independent working man. You, the man who has a family. The man who works out all the time or the man who doesn't work out at all and wants to. This book is about taking care of your body, the machine. It exists solely to help men live strong and healthy lives with strong healthy bodies.

Stretching, as we have seen throughout this guide, is an easy-to-start and easy-to-achieve form of exercise. It yields effective results equal to regular strength and endurance training with little to no effort. Understanding what exactly stretching is and the wide range of benefits it has for anyone, especially senior citizens, is crucial. Hopefully, you have come to understand the physical side of stretching and the mental side in equal measure.

There then remains no excuse to not have and maintain a physically fit and healthy body as we age, and in truth, the same goes for every person out there. In this guide, we've gone over why stretching is an excellent choice of exercise for senior citizens. We focused on how it benefits men in detail and how to tackle it if you're just starting. Finally, we found a range of different exercises to focus on different important areas of our bodies.

Incorporating a daily stretching routine in your life has never been easier than with the correct use and understanding of this guide. Stretching does not require a gym membership, nor does it require a lot of equipment. It can be done anywhere and at any time. Making it an enjoyable experience through music, practicing with friends, or taking it into nature and exercising in the park.

Stretching for men seems to be a no-brainer. Being mindful while practicing stretching also increases our mental capacity to add to the physical benefits of the exercise.

That said, as with any type of exercise, keeping safety in mind is always important. Following the guidelines in this book and consulting with your doctor will ensure successful and beneficial stretching. Be persistent in practicing, using the correct techniques, and maintaining focus; the long-term results are worth it. Whether they be in the form of more flexibility, mobility, or a general range of motion, the benefits are there and easy to achieve.

The information I have provided to you in this book is from my own experience as well as a high amount of research on the stretching topic. I wanted to be able to only give you the best recommendations and suggestions out there. With this information, followed by the letter, you should be able to accomplish the maximum flexibility permitted by your body structure. While at the same time developing your strength.

Finally, if you enjoyed reading this book or have any feedback suggestions, then I would kindly ask you to leave a review behind on Amazon. Should you have suggestions for a subject in the future that you want to explore further, please let me know through the review button as well. It would be greatly appreciated by the community.

Printed in Great Britain
by Amazon